TIPS FOR HAPPINESS
In The Shadow of
CANCER

Can I? *"I Can...* *...I will"*

TIPS FOR HAPPINESS In The Shadow of CANCER

Can I? "I Can... ...I will"

Dr. Meenu Walia

Message

Shri. J.P. Nadda

Hon'ble Minister of Health & Family Welfare,
Govt. of India

Foreword

Ms. Manisha Koirala

Film Actress & Cancer Warrior

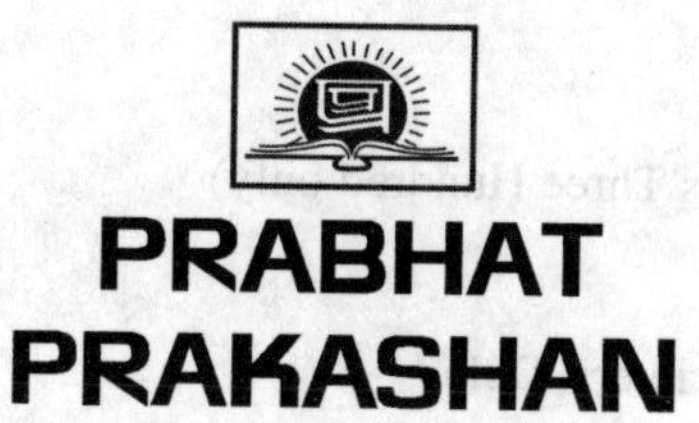

PRABHAT
PRAKASHAN

Published by
PRABHAT PAPERBACKS
An imprint of Prabhat Prakashan Pvt. Ltd.
4/19 Asaf Ali Road,
New Delhi-110 002 (INDIA)
e-mail: prabhatbooks@gmail.com

ISBN 978-93-5186-626-8
TIPS FOR HAPPINESS
IN THE SHADOW OF CANCER
by Dr. Meenu Walia

Cover Image
Ms. Parimita Sahoo

Edition
2023

Price
₹ 300.00 (Rupees Three Hundred only)

Printed at
R-Tech Offset Printers, Delhi

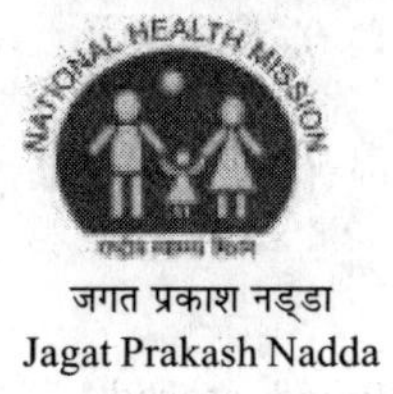

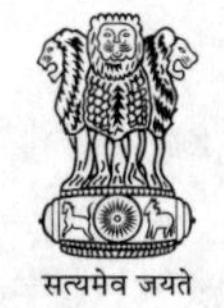

सत्यमेव जयते

स्वास्थ्य एवं परिवार कल्याण मंत्री
भारत सरकार
Minister of Health & Family Welfare
Government of India

जगत प्रकाश नड्डा
Jagat Prakash Nadda

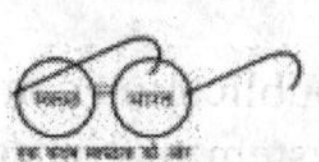

Message

Dr. Meenu Walia, has dedicated several years of her life treating cancer patients and working closely with patients' family and relatives. From the years of experience in her field and her personal experience gained by interacting with the patients and their families, Dr. Walia has tried to put her thoughts and experience together to bring awareness to the society in the form of this book.

The book 'Tips for Happiness: In the Shadow of Cancer' is a well presented book. It provides motivation not just for a cancer patient but for anyone in general.

The book is well written and will surely help the patients and their close ones gain courage, strength and motivation in their fight against the disease.

The true stories of the victims of this disease and the quotes cited in the book touch one's heart. They are inspiring and motivating. I wish all the best to Dr. Meenu Walia for these efforts.

(Jagat Prakash Nadda)

348, ए-स्कंध, निर्माण भवन, नई दिल्ली-110011
348, A-Wing, Nirman Bhawan, New Delhi 110011
Tele.: (O) +91-11-23061661, 23061751 Telefax: 23062358, 23061648
E-mail: hfwminister@gov.in

Jagat Prakash Nadda

Minister of Health & Family Welfare
Government of India

Message

Dr. Meenu Walia has dedicated several years of her life treating cancer patients and working closely with them. [illegible] expertise in her field and her personal experience gained by interacting with the patients and their families, Dr. Walia has tried to put her thoughts and experience together to bring awareness to the society in the form of this book.

The book 'Tips for Happiness: In the Shadow of Cancer' is a well presented book. It provides motivation not just for a cancer patient but for anyone in general. The book is well written and will surely help the patients and their close ones gain courage, strength and motivation in their fight against the disease.

The true stories of the victims of this disease and the quotes quoted in the book touch one's heart. They are inspiring and motivating. I wish all the best to Dr. Meenu Walia for these efforts.

(Jagat Prakash Nadda)

348, A-Wing, Nirman Bhawan, New Delhi-110011
Tele: (O) +91-11-23061661, 23061751 Telefax: 23062358, 23061648
E-mail: hfwminister@gov.in

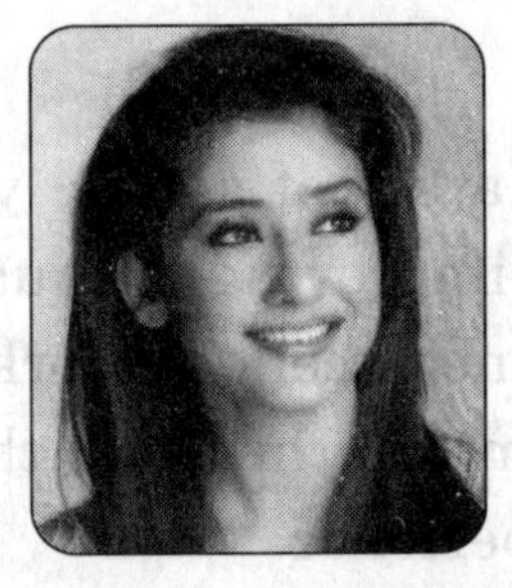

Foreword

The book 'Tips for Happiness: In the Shadow of Cancer' is intended not only for people whose lives have been stricken by this dreadful disease but for anyone who either himself or herself or whose near and dear one is going through a troubled phase in life.

It is a step by step handbook to attain control over life during difficult times and emerge as a winner.

Who else could know more about the deadly affliction than the author Dr. Meenu Walia. Watching her closely in the battle field against Cancer has been a revelation. Her untiring efforts, be it in the clinical field dealing with her patients for endless hours in the hospital, or creating awareness in the community, leading the screening programs on weekends, delivering talks, speak about the vengeance with which she has decided to take the fight to the other camp.

Dr. Walia has beautifully crafted a wonderful

book revealing a set of simple yet surprisingly potent ideas for improving the quality of anyone's life. She has done excellent work in putting the pearls of wisdom together over the thread of her professional experience.

Her years of experience as a cancer specialist has helped her write a very meaningful and practical book for anybody suffering from the disease.

Flipping through the pages, one can see that it addresses every possible issue associated with Cancer, right from diagnosis to cure and thereafter. It touches upon the vulnerability of the patient as he is diagnosed, moves on to stress on the need to immediately get on with the treatment once diagnosed, the need to maintain continuity of the treatment preferably in the hands of one constant team of consultants, the diet to be followed, harnessing the mental strengths to keep the fight going. A really handy guide for those looking for answers to their endless questions and conflicts.

The book also serves as a guide to the close relatives of the patients, addresses even the distant relatives and friends of those afflicted. The personal accounts of the survivors giving their own stories of their victories and tribulations are inspiring indeed.

Last but not the least inspiring quotes generously peppered around the pages are a delight to read.

There are many who fight their own battles, inspired are those who fight other's battle like their own. Blessed are those who fight during the day, and heal during the night so that the fight can go on.

—Manisha Koirala

Bollywood Actress &
Cancer Warrior

Mumbai
09.01.2016

Acknowledgement

'Thank you' is just a word but the implications are worthy enough. I would like to gather up words and thank 'The Almighty' for blessing me with all what I have today and what all I had accomplished in the past.

I am really grateful to Mr. Ganga Kumar who conceptualized the idea of this book and pushed me to a momentum where I decided to put my experience into words. He had a tough time getting me to work on it (after months of pursuance).

Family has always been a source of inspiration to me. My husband Harminder, who has been of immense help in motivating me and being the serene listener, uncomplainingly undergoing the ordeal of reviewing the book. Special thanks to my son Praneet for the innocent suggestions (and also for not disturbing me). My Father, Mr G.S. Walia finds a special mention in this for his unshakeable faith in my abilities.

Tonnes of thanks to Dr. Abrar and Mr. Sanjay for their valuable time and inputs. Without their support and help, this book would not have been possible.

"You never know how strong you are until being strong is the only choice you have"

—Cayla Mills

I am indebted to all my patients, who have been 'heroes' in so many ways. Many of their simple words of wisdom have stayed with me and have been used by me in writing this book.

Introduction

One can never forget the day, the exact moment when he/she is diagnosed with cancer. For almost everybody, it is a life-changing experience. This book intends to serve as a guide to bounce back in life and get up on your feet, as it was the way earlier.

I came across many people, who I have seen crying on the day of diagnosis and with tears of joy after completing the treatment. This is a depiction of the rollercoaster of emotions which I have witnessed and made me feel connected to my patients. We all learn from our mistakes but wise are those who learn from others' mistakes. This book is an effort to encompass the misconceptions, fears, social stigma, course of treatment and ultimately how to deal with the situations to resurface as a winner. I am not a philosopher or a saint or an expert about life. All what I could say in this book is, what I have been taught by the patients. Most patients that I came across had developed their own simple ways to overcome the problems and move on. Many of their simple words of wisdom have stayed with me and have been used by me in writing this book. The success stories are to instill your inner self with never ending inspiration so that even if you get weak at any point of time in life, the success stories and advices may help you pull up your socks and start running towards victory. The success stories are to show you how to deal with the situations, shut yourself off from despair and how to face the discouragements of the world.

Contents

Chapter 1

The Word Cancer and Denial

> *"Even as your body betrays you,*
> *your mind denies it"*
> **—Sara Gruen**

In my practice of 21 years, I have seen people facing the gloomy diagnosis – the evil Cancer and have seen them undergo so much of emotional, financial and health related crisis that I have no other means of comparison than using 5 stages of death as described by Kubler – Ross. The very first stage is described as denial. The very first time when I look into a new patient's eyes, the very eye contact says it all, it says how the patient is going to handle the big news. When I saw Revati for the first time in OPD, she was all scared for the lump in her breast. After clinical examination, I was quite certain that the lump was something else than a benign mass. She is a mid-thirties female with an educated background. Probably she had done all the Google research on the breast lumps. Two situations are the most critical for me to handle; breaking the news and discussing the prognosis. I looked into her eyes and told her to get the biopsy done. She had millions of questions in her mind. I was hoping myself to be wrong because I feared for something bad ahead – though manageable. Five days passed by and Revati came with her reports. Biopsy reports were positive for cancer. I could see the doubts in her eyes regarding the reports and the denial was very much clear from her words and body language. One by one phrases "this can't be", "there must be some mistake", "the samples must have gotten mixed up" and "take another biopsy" kept echoing in the room.

I made Revati come to a situation where she was able to understand my words. For her satisfaction, the biopsy sample was rechecked but in vain. It didn't change anything in diagnosis. And this wasn't for the first time that I was seeing such kind of emotional reactions. But what I told her, was something I usually tell everyone who comes to me with similar problems.

Yes, human error is possible but most pathologists take utmost care before pronouncing the 'malignancy' report. When, in doubt, it is easier for a pathologist to write 'inconclusive' than to give the diagnosis.

Tips to handle denial:

1. **Gather knowledge** – read all kinds of information regarding your condition, what you are terrified of. But do not waste too much time in gathering information as delay may prove further detrimental and disastrous.
2. **Consult a doctor** – seek medical advice from a specialist in this field if you suspect

anything wrong. If you are not convinced, then do not hesitate to seek a second opinion.

3. If in doubt, request your doctor / pathologist to **review the reports**.

□

> *I feel that as long as you're honest, you have the opportunity to grow. It's when you shut down, go into denial, and try to start hiding things from yourself and others, that's when you lock in certain behaviours and attitudes that keep you stuck.*
>
> **—Tracy McMillan**

Chapter 2

Why Me?

> *"If I were to say 'God why me?' about the bad things, then I should have said 'God why me?' about the good things that happened in my life."*
>
> **—Arthur Ashe**

Sushma had been waiting outside my OPD since 8 am (though my OPD timings were from 9 am onwards). I reached my OPD on my scheduled time and saw her waiting anxiously. She came in the room and the very look on her face had a self explained anger. This anger towards the disease, the life, and just everyone else. This is again one stage where people are not in a situation to understand the necessary steps to be taken further, because they are still not able to absorb the diagnosis. Her barrage of questions were neither slowing down nor stopping. ***"Why me?", "Who is to blame?", "What wrong did I do to get this disease?", "Why is God punishing me?"*** and so on. After seeing so many patients, I can fairly understand the practical implications of the diagnosis. Ill effects have not come yet. They are to follow. Sushma's husband had a tough time dealing with her emotions. We had to counsel her regarding self-created illusion of imminent death, after making her understand that it is not the end of the world. Her cancer was in early stage and after she underwent surgery, the relief which was quite evident from her smile was the best reward I could imagine of. This is not just one person's story, we have thousands of Sushma, facing the trouble – some take it as a challenge and some take it as a punishment from destiny. Those who take it as challenge and fight against all odds, have the winner's smile.

Almost everybody suffers from this "Why me" syndrome. If you too face it, you are not alone!

Tips to handle "Why me?" syndrome:

1. **Don't try to find answers of "Why Me?" syndrome**. Answers probably don't exist.
2. **Dealing with anger** – It is a natural human behaviour to be angry towards adversities which you can't change. Take a moment to realize that with adversities, come their solutions. With mind clouded with anger, we tend to miss the solutions that are just around the corner. Take control of your emotions because just the diagnosis isn't the end of the world.
3. **No more "why me"** – Get out of the phase as soon as possible because there is no end to these questions. Remember that Universe doesn't give you what you ask for with your thoughts; it gives you what you demand with your actions.
4. **Remember, cancer is an accident which can happen to anyone**.
5. **Accept the diagnosis.**

6. **Denial will not help,** nor will delay in treatment.

7. **Remember** – the best time to plant a tree was 20 years ago. The next best time is 'Now'.

ACT NOW. DO NOT WASTE TIME.
SEEK HELP. DO NOT PANIC

□

> *"God give me courage to change the things I can and strength to accept the things I cannot."*
>
> **—Anonymous**

Chapter 3
Vanquishing Fear

> *"It is better by noble boldness to run the risk of being subject to half of the evils we anticipate, than to remain in cowardly listlessness for fear of what may happen"*
>
> **—Herodotus**

I was sitting in my OPD chamber, explaining the treatment options to a new patient. The patient was given the option of chemotherapy during the last visit. The patient and the attendants had come back to discuss again the side-effects of chemotherapy which were explained last time. After about half an hour of counselling and explanation of side-effects the patient and the attendants still had that perplexed look, while leaving the room. The next patient Kalawati, who was a very old patient of mine, now on follow-up entered with an exhausted look on her face. When she and her husband looked at me with those complaining eyes, I knew their wait had been too long. The previous patient had taken a lot of time. I looked at them and tried to yield an explanation "***a new patient...... still taking time to accept the side-effects of treatment and trying to take decision***"

"***Oh! This patient intends crossing the river without entering the water".*** With a chuckle, Kalawati added ***"May be he is hoping for the river to dry-up***". Her simple words struck me and stayed with me.

Invariably, majority of the cancer patients are scared. There is a fear about everything – fear of cancer as well as fear of the ordeal of the treatment.

Things we understand are easy to handle. But what about the things we don't understand? We either close our eyes towards them or we develop a fear towards them. Everybody is scared of the big 'C'. Ignorance about the disease and the uncertainty about future can build into enormous fear.

Though there has been a lot of research on cancer, there has been no social awareness or a very little social awareness regarding the evil. For a common man, the word Cancer is synonymous with death. Many people still fear that 'Cancer = Death'. The fear society has knit around cancer and its treatment, which is generally baseless, makes a patient think that he is inching towards an imminent death. This society generated sentence is the primal fear that grips the patient and keeps on stinging him till he loses inner strength. But the fact is that, most cancers are treatable. If things have to go wrong, then even malaria or tuberculosis can kill a person. Although uncertainty about the outcomes may be there but treatment is available for majority of cancers. Remember one thing that "if victory is certain, even a coward can fight but real warrior is the one who keeps fighting despite the uncertain outcome". One day, we all have to perish, but what matters is how we perish. There is nothing worse than succumbing to your own fears.

Tips to cope up with fear:

1. **Does fear yield results**? Ask yourself, what did you do when you had exam next morning? Didn't you study instead of being scared and crying on the pillow? Would you have cleared the exam, if you would be sobbing the entire time? No! Then why sobbing now? Hide the tears of fear and use it later as tears of joy after victory.

2. **Uncertainty yields fear**. Talk to your doctor. Ask questions. Try to get clear answers.

3. **Ask your doctor** to guide you to the right source of information.

4. **Talk** to another patient or better, a survivor.

5. **Join a support group**. As understanding of disease sets in, insecurities and fear will recede.

6. **Seek help** – It is not a matter of shame to seek help. This help can come from your family, friends or even your counselor. Yes

counselor, who can be a psychiatrist; who can train you to cope up with your fears.

7. **Give all, than giving up** – We all have a fighter in us, but due to fear of unforeseen consequences we back down and give up even before gearing up for the fight.

□

> *"You are only afraid if you are not in harmony with yourself. People are afraid because they have never owned up to themselves".*
>
> **—Hermann Hesse**

Chapter 4

Hope is Always Around the Corner

"You are only afraid if you are not in harmony with yourself. People are afraid because they have never owned up to themselves."

—Hermann Hesse

Chapter 4

Hope is Always Around the Corner

"Hold fast to dreams, for if dreams die life is a broken-winged bird that cannot fly."

—Langston Hughes

"There is no medicine like hope, no incentive so great and no tonic so powerful as expectation of something tomorrow."

I had reached the OPD earlier that day. Mid-January was the month and it was chilling cold outside. I had time to sip a cup of tea before the rush of OPD started. Sipping the hot tea, I asked Kavita, my OPD nurse, to read over the list of appointments for the day. She uttered the name of Beena. I had three patients by the name of Beena receiving treatment at that point of time. I casually asked her – 'which Beena' is this, expecting she would tell the diagnosis. "The one who always comes in a new dress and that bright lipstick" came the prompt reply. She went on to murmur "I wonder how these patients get time to dress up so nicely and put make-up, in spite of being sick." The comment made me acknowledge the fact that yes, that particular patient of mine always made that extra effort to dress-up nicely. That day, when Beena walked into my OPD, I complimented her on her dress and asked her how she always managed to dress-up so nicely. Her answer was not what I was expecting "The idea of every chemotherapy session makes me feel low and run down. Putting up a nice dress just cheers me up".

A pretty dress, a string of pearls, a bright lip shade are all trivial material things. But these are probably the ways, some of the patients interact with the world outside and keep their morale high. They probably tell the world that they have HOPE. Sometimes, the only thing that you have left is hope. "Hope that tomorrow will hurt little less than yesterday."

Tips to keep hope alive:

1. **Hold on to faith**. Have faith in yourself. If you can't, then have faith in those who have faith in you.
2. **Seek religious help**.
3. **Plan a trip** after completion of every segment of treatment. You have something to look forward to.
4. **Connect** with your good memories.
5. **Remember** – what appears as the end today is probably just a bend. Keep going.

Upanishads say 'Chairaveti, chairaveti'. It means "go on, go on. Do not halt". Do not stagnate, keep going on!

□

"The tragedy of life is not death, but what we let die inside of us while we live."

—Norman Cousins

Chapter 5

Get Set Go

Chapter 5

Get Set Go

> *"The hardest step for a runner is the first one out of the front door."*
>
> **—Anonymous**

"Madam, a patient is waiting for you in OPD" informed Azad my-OPD coordinator.

'Who?' I asked, while on ward rounds.

"Mr Suresh, last seen by us on 12th January for complaints of cough and chest pain."

"Ok, collect his reports and tell him that I'm coming".

Hurrying to OPD after completing my rounds, I just recalled about him. He came to me for complaints of chest pain and cough. But wasn't that 5 months back? May be, he started his treatment at some other centre. All my assumptions were about to be pulverized in next 5 minutes. A glance of his lemony yellow turned eyes made me sigh and I whispered to myself ***'oh dear lord'.***

"Where were you Suresh ji for all these months?" I asked him.

"Madam ji, we thought of getting the reports reconfirmed."

"For so long?" I asked,controlling my anger on his laid back attitude.

"Now I am ready for the treatment, I did not take any treatment. Till now I wanted to be sure of the disease. Now I am sure, please treat me."

Shocked at his reply, I asked ***"what? No treatment till now?"***

'Yes' he said.

Looking at his reports, I figured out the entire story. Majority of the papers had OPD prescriptions of so many doctors, from north to south! It took him 5 months to be sure of the disease. Initially, which was a curable disease, his lack of decision-making and delay made it an incurable one. His prolonged medical shopping has brought this doom upon him and his family. Now he has developed liver metastases with jaundice which rendered him unfit for any anti-cancer treatment. The news was heartbreaking for the entire family. But there are circumstances where you can't do anything. But what was more heartbreaking was that these circumstances were brought upon by the patient himself and his family and could have been avoided with timely treatment. A treatable situation was made terminal because of lack of sense of urgency. He ultimately lost his battle to cancer even before he could draw out his sword and make a blow.

I have seen many people visiting doctors to doctors and hospital to hospital, not realizing the importance of 'Time'. Taking second opinion is fine but fourth, fifth, sixth..... for how long? This series of opinions will never stop and at the end of the day, you will realize that you were sleeping at the edge of the volcano, assuming that you still have time. Remember, every case is a different case and every human body is different. In medicine, 2 + 2 may we always be 4. The disease can progress at any pace which nobody can predict. So don't waste time!

Tips to Get Set and Go

1. **Be quick in taking decisions** – Don't be just quick in taking decisions, be wise too. Not every doctor has the same expertise and not all hospitals are well equipped for the specialized treatment. This is where friends and family can be of great help. Scout them to find suitable doctor, suitable hospital. Do not waste too much time in medical shopping! Get moving and don't panic. If you are not moving, you will never be able to walk down the lane.
2. **Selecting right Doctor** – Look for a qualified and experienced Oncologist. Check your comfort level with the doctor.
3. **Selecting the right Hospital** – This is the 2nd most important factor to be considered after doctor. Look for the hospital which has all the departments and

facilities pertaining to Medical, Surgical and Radiation Oncology. Don't be an island jumper by selecting different doctors and hospitals for different phases of treatment as this may hamper the original plan of the treatment.

□

"I think failure is nothing more than life's way of nudging you that you are off course. My attitude to failure is not attached to outcome, but in not trying at all."

—Sara Blakely

Chapter 6

Be Your Own Filter... Block That Noise

> *"And it is easy to believe you are not good enough if you listen to everybody else."*
>
> **—Mackenzie Astin**

There will be endless bombardment of ideas, advices, theories and medical bullying thrown on you. There will be continuous over-flow of information on what to do and what not to do. You talk or you don't talk – advices pour in. You sit on internet and the flood of information leaves you more confused and drained. For a patient, who is over burdened with information, it actually causes negative physical, mental, emotional and social impacts. For this type of situation a British psychologist, Lewis, coined the phrase ***information fatigue syndrome***. Gaining information more than required may result into *analysis paralysis* and making it increasingly difficult to identify and select relevant information. In this environment of continuous bombardment of information, it is hard to make decisions and easy to get depressed, anxious and exhausted.

Tips to tackle:

1. **Sit back and take a deep breath**. Clear that clutter.
2. **Take an informed decision**
   - Once you have chosen a hospital and doctor, remember your doctor is your best source of information. Ask your doctor-

which medical internet site gives authenticated information, that you should follow.

- In a similar fashion – just pick up one or maximum of two acquaintances who can guide you.

Important criteria of selecting your advisors should be:

- Advisor is a positive personality.
- He or she is either a survivor/a close caretaker of a cancer patient.

□

> *"Keep what is worth keeping; with breath of kindness, blow rest away."*
>
> **—Dinah M Craik**

Chapter 7

Coping with the Treatment

> *"Sometimes you don't realize your own strength until you come face to face with your greatest weakness."*
>
> **—Susan Gale**

Initiating the treatment is not the difficult part. What is more challenging, is to complete the treatment, despite facing side effects. Nobody else knows it better than Mrs. Roma. She is on treatment for past 5-6 years and till date, manages the side effects quite well. She has stage IV cancer and lives on to share her experience with us. Most of the people see marks of chemotherapy as a matter of embarrassment. But I recall the tribes of hunters/ warriors who carry the scars of struggle proudly and consider it their sign of triumph. It is your battle and these are your scars of victory. Then why do you have to be ashamed of it?

Tips to Cope Up With the Treatment

1. **Make a list of Do's and Don'ts** – Take help of your Doctor and prepare a list of what is to be avoided during the treatment and what all is permitted. The list can contain all sorts of information from what kind of fabric to be worn and even your personal habits. If you can't consult your doctor, take help of authentic websites, booklets and reading materials and atleast get it approved by your treating doctor.
2. **Mark your calendar** and set up reminders for your appointments.

3. **Allocate responsibilities** – Take help of your family members regarding your needs and treatment-related tasks. You might not be a very good cook, or might not be a tech-savvy or even have a forgetful mind. Someone who is good at cooking can take up responsibility of your diet during treatment; someone who is tech-savvy can use calendar apps to mark dates of your chemotherapy and appointments and setup alerts accordingly. Some family member might be a fitness freak who can help you with yoga or light exercise. If resources are to be utilized wisely, things can be managed quite easily.

4. **Ask for a checklist from your doctor or hospital:** (Most hospitals have checklists and you can request one) regarding your checkups and treatment along with precautions.

5. **Make your questionnaire**: You may have hundreds of questions dwelling in your mind while you are at home, but tend to forget half of them inside the doctor's chamber. Write down your queries in a small pocket diary and ask your doctor on the next visit.

6. **Emergency:** You should know when to seek emergency medical attention and whom to contact. Keep emergency contact numbers handy for easy accessibility.

7. **Diet:** Pay special attention to your diet. Take help of a dietician, if required.

8. **Take adequate sleep** – A proper night's sleep especially between 11 pm and 7 am will help you heal, minimum 8 hours of sleep is required. Restful sleep also stimulates your regenerative abilities. If possible, take a nap in afternoon and replenish your energy levels.

9. **Hide it or Flaunt it** – Treatment may leave behind marks of identification which might make you stand out from the crowd. For example, some chemotherapies leave people bald and some cause nail discoloration. Simple tweaks may help you not to feel inferior to others in terms of looks. You can use wigs, caps or scarves to hide your baldness. Women can use nail paints to hide discolored nails, which they may find a matter of embarrassment. Mrs. Vidhi is one such inspiration, who lost her hair during treatment. Now she doesn't feel ashamed of it, rather she has made her 'Bald look' – her style statement.

10. **Find your own 'De-Stress recipe'** – Engage in activities that relax you.
    (a) Yoga
    (b) Meditation
    (c) Listening to music
    (d) Watching a movie
    (e) Gardening
    (f) Reading a book
    (g) Painting
    (h) Getting a spa...... the list is endless

11. **Know your limits:** Don't be over enthusiastic with extra energy you get by motivation. As they say, overcooking the curry leaves a burnt taste. So, know your limits.

□

> *"Life is not what it's supposed to be. It's what it is. The way you cope with it, is what makes the difference."*
>
> **—Virginia Satir**

Chapter 8

Quitting is Never an Option

"Pain is temporary. Quitting lasts forever"....

—Lance Armstrong

"Cancer is only going to be a chapter in my life and not the whole story"....

—Joe Wasser

Amod who appeared numb and disheveled during our first two meetings, was a different person when he walked into the OPD the third time. Amod had presented to me with huge abdominal lump, which had already been biopsied outside and diagnosed as cancer. After the initial steps of diagnosis confirmation and staging work-up, I had planned to start chemotherapy that day. As is common – everybody wants to sit and discuss the disease and the side effects of chemotherapy. I could make out from Nalini's (patient's wife) face that she was being haunted by the same questions and wanted to discuss the same. As soon as, I pulled my writing pad and opened my mouth trying to explain the side-effects, I was interrupted by a very calm, composed Amod. He said "doctor sahab, No I don't want to know the side effects nor what chances I have. I know only one thing – medicines has really revolutionized and cures are available". I just want to start treatment.

That day and for days after, Amod had silenced both me and his wife. The chemotherapy began that day and the sessions continued. Today, more than ten years have passed since that day and Amod still visits me with his wife. Every time I see him, his words still echo. I salute his spirit and wonder – is that the reason that even a decade later, he stays in complete remission and free of disease.

Time and again, it has been scientifically proven that patients who maintain a positive attitude do better.

Tips to be positive:

1. Make a **conscious decision** to stay away from negative people.
2. Have your own collection of **positive books.**
3. Everytime you come across a **positive quote**, make a note. Write it somewhere where you can see it often, whether on the door, almirah or bathroom mirror.
4. Make your own collage of **positive memories**. Like, pictures of your marriage, the first gift you gave your parents, the first gift your daughter gave you... etc. etc.

□

> *"Age wrinkles the body,*
> *quitting wrinkles the soul"*
> **—Douglas Mc Arthur**

Chapter 9

Cancer Fighting Kitchen

Chapter 9

Cancer Fighting Kitchen

> *"The food you eat can be either the safest and the most powerful form of medicine or the slowest form of poison."*
>
> **—Ann Wigmore**

Healthy Platter: Prevent Cancer

Focus on cancer-fighting fruits and vegetables:

- Diets, high in fruit may lower the risk of stomach and lung cancer.
- Eating vegetables containing carotenoids, such as carrots, may reduce the risk of lung, mouth, pharynx, and larynx cancers.
- Diets high in non-starchy vegetables, such as broccoli, spinach, and beans, may help protect against stomach and esophageal cancer.
- Eating oranges, berries, peas, capsicum, dark leafy greens and other foods high in vitamin C may also protect against esophageal cancer.
- Lycopene rich fruits and vegetables, such as tomatoes, guava, and watermelon, may lower the risk of prostate cancer.

Fight cancer with fiber:

Eating a diet high in fiber may help prevent colorectal cancer and other common digestive system cancers, including stomach, mouth, and pharynx.

It also prevents constipation by adding bulk of food.

Fiber is found in fruits, vegetables, and whole

grains. In general, the more natural and unprocessed the food, the higher it is in fiber. There is no fiber in meat, dairy, sugar, or 'white' foods like white bread, white rice, and pastries.

- Use brown rice instead of white rice.
- Substitute whole-grain bread for white bread or multigrain bread over white bread.
- Choose a bran muffin over a croissant or pastry.
- Snack on popcorn instead of potato chips or dry fruits would be even healthier.
- Enjoy steamed carrots, celery, or bell peppers with a salsa, low fat salad dressing or lemon juices, instead of chips and a sour cream dip.
- Use beans instead of ground meat in sandwiches, pakoras and even burgers (bean burgers can taste great).

Aqua Magic:-Fiber absorbs water so the more fiber you add to your diet, the more fluids you should drink. Water is also essential for fighting cancer. It stimulates the immune system, removes waste and toxins, and transports nutrients to all of your organs.

Cut down on meat: – High meat diet or meat rich diet has a toll on health if you have a sedentary lifestyle. Moreover, red meat has been linked to gut cancer. You can cut down your cancer risk substantially by reducing the amount of animal-based products you eat and by choosing healthier meats.

- **Keep meat to a minimum** Try to keep the total amount of meat in your diet not more than fifteen percent of your total calories. Ten percent is even better.
- **Eat red meat occasionally.** Red meat is high in saturated fat, so eat it sparingly. Better to avoid it.
- **Reduce the portion size of meat in each meal.** The portion should be able to fit in the palm of your hand.
- **Use meat as a flavouring or a side, not the main focus of a meal.** You can use a little bit of meat to add flavour or texture to your food, rather than using it as the main element.
- **Add beans** and other plant-based protein sources to your meals.
- **Choose leaner meats,** such as fish, chicken, or turkey.
- **Avoid processed meats** such as hotdogs, sausage, and salami, ready to eat meat products.
- **Select organic meat. If you have access to it.** Organic livestock must have access to the outdoors and be given organic feed, free of GMOs*. They may not be given

*GMO (Genetically Modified Organisms) refers to any food product that has been altered at the gene level.

antibiotics, growth hormones, or any animal-by-products.

Choose your fats wisely

Eating a diet high in fat increases your risk for many types of cancer and not just cancer, it poses risk of cholesterol issues. But cutting out fat entirely isn't the answer, either. In fact, some types of fat may actually protect against cancer and cholesterol issues. The trick is to choose your fats wisely and eat them in moderation.

How to decide:-Fats solid at room temperature are considered bad for you.

- **Fats that increase cancer risk** – The two most damaging fats are saturated fats and trans fats. Saturated fats are found mainly in animal products such as red meat, whole milk dairy products,. Trans fats, also called partially hydrogenated oils, are created by adding hydrogen to liquid vegetable oils to make them more solid and less likely to spoil—which is very good for food manufacturers, and very bad for you.
- **Fats that decrease cancer risk** – The best fats are unsaturated fats, which come from plant sources and are liquid at room temperature. Primary sources include olive oil, canola oil, nuts, and avocados. Also focus on omega-3 fatty acids, which fight

inflammation and support brain and heart health. Good sources include cod liver oil (available in capsule form) salmon, tuna and flaxseeds.

Prepare your food in healthy ways:

Choosing healthy food is not the only important factor. It also matters how you prepare and store your food. The way you cook your food can either be a healthy platter or health splatter.

Boosting the cancer-fighting benefits of food

Here are a few tips that will help you get all the benefits from eating those great cancer-fighting foods, such as fruit and vegetables:

- **Eat at least some raw fruits and vegetables.** These have the highest amounts of vitamins and minerals, although cooking some vegetables can make the vitamins more available for our body to use.
- **When cooking vegetables, steam until just tender, using a small amount of water.** This preserves more of the vitamins. Overcooking vegetables removes many of the vitamins and minerals. If you do boil vegetables, use the cooking water in a soup

or another dish to ensure you're getting all the vitamins.

- **Wash all fruits and vegetables.** Use a vegetable brush for washing. Washing does not eliminate all pesticide residues, but will reduce it. Choose organic produce if possible, grown without the use of pesticides or GMOs.
- **Flavour food with immune-boosting herbs and spices.** Garlic, ginger, and curry powder not only add flavour, but they add a cancer-fighting punch of valuable nutrients. Other good choices include turmeric, basil, rosemary, and coriander. Use them in soups, salads, casseroles, or any other dish.
- **Use salad dressing made by olive oils instead of plain salad.** This enhances the taste as well as nutritive values.

Tips for avoiding carcinogens

Carcinogens are cancer-causing substances found in food. Carcinogens can form during the cooking or preserving process—mostly in relation to meat—and as foods start to spoil. Examples of foods that have carcinogens are cured, dried, and preserved meats (e.g. bacon, sausage, burned or charred meats; smoked foods; and foods that have become moldy. Here are some ways reduce your exposure to carcinogens:

- **Do not cook oils on high heat.** Low-heat cooking or baking (less than 240 degrees) prevents oils or fats from turning carcinogenic. Instead of deep-frying, pan-frying, and sautéing, opt for healthier methods such as baking, boiling, steaming, or broiling.
- **Go easy on the barbecue.** Burning or charring meats creates carcinogenic substances. If you do choose to barbecue, don't overcook the meat and be sure to cook at the proper temperature (not too hot) or pre-tenderise by pressure cooking and then grilling reduces charring of food.
- **Store oils in a cool dark place in airtight containers,** as they quickly become rancid when exposed to heat, light, and air.
- **Choose fresh meats** instead of cured, dried, preserved, or smoked meats.
- **Avoid foods that look or smell moldy,** as they are likely to contain aflatoxin, a strong carcinogen. Aflatoxin is most commonly found on moldy peanuts. Nuts will stay fresh longer if kept in the refrigerator or freezer. Better would be salt roasting of nuts.

- **Be careful what you put in the microwave.** Use waxed paper rather than plastic wrap to cover your food in the microwave. And always use microwave-safe containers. Use microwave-safe glass wares instead of plastic containers.

Dietary tips for patients on therapy

Cancer often drains people's energies, moods and thoughts. Simple tweaks in the diet and dietary habits can replenish your energy levels. Consult your doctor and dietician regarding the Do's and Don'ts of diet. Following tips may further benefit you, though.

1. Food Safety

Food safety is a special concern to cancer patients.

A. Wash hands thoroughly before eating and before food preparations.

B. Wash hands before food preparation, and wash fruits and vegetables thoroughly before eating.

C. Handle raw meats with care. Keep it away from cooked foods.

D. Cook meat/poultry/fish thoroughly.

E. Use pasteurized/boiled milk.

F. If eating away from home, avoid salads,

sushi, and raw/undercooked meats and eggs.

G. Take particular care with drinking water.

2. Preventing Nausea:

Hunger prolongs nausea. Eat small, frequent meals. Enjoy snacks between the meals.

Keep up fluid intake – sip your drink slowly. You may find it helpful to freeze limejuice or other juice, and suck on the frozen bits. Once the worst of nausea has passed, try a ginger ale, weak tea or green tea, popsicles, clear broth and soup.

3. How to tolerate smell of Food:

People have an altered sense of smell while on chemotherapy.

How to handle that? Simple solution is avoid pungent smelling ingredients. Sometimes fragrant ingredients have to be eliminated too.

Eg. – Avoid Ginger – garlic

- Avoid strong smelling food like sea food.
- Avoid stuffs like Garam Masala, Cardamom, cinnamon etc.

4. Lost Appetite:

To cope up with loss of appetite or unable to tolerate heavy meals – Eat energy rich, small and frequent meals. Include homemade snacks in your diet if you are craving for short eats.

- Take dry freshly salt roasted dry fruits for the inter meal cravings.
- Take good quality branded chocolates as they are a good source of energy.

5. Coping up with Chemotherapy induced constipation:

- Include fiber rich food into your diet.
- Breakfast: Make a sweet porridge with Milk, Oatmeat and sugar. Apart from providing nutrition, it will help fight constipation too. Adding nutrition supplements while cooking further reinforces nutrition.
- Drink plenty of water:-use pre boiled and cooled filtered water.

6. If you are more of a meat lover:

- Avoid fish/ sea food if you can't tolerate the smell while on chemo.
- Avoid red meat as it is a little hard to digest and induces constipation.
- Eat chicken – freshly cut and properly cooked, not the frozen ones.
- Use olive oil while preparing meat dishes as it eliminates odour and packs nutrition.
- If you have access to extra virgin olive oil, use it for your cooking purpose.

7. Sore mouth or Difficulty in swallowing

You may have a sore mouth or difficulty in swallowing food:

A. Try smooth or blended foods, or creamy consistency.

B. Avoid foods that sting your mouth like acidic fruit (pineapple), or spicy and salty foods.

C. Avoid rough crunchy foods like hard toast and nuts.

D. Try drinking through a straw.

E. Pay special attention to mouth hygiene to prevent infection and tooth decay.

F. Use a gentle mouthwash after meals.

8. For a Dry Mouth

A. Take fluids with your meal.

B. Suck on chips of ice. They also stimulate flow of saliva.

C. Add gravy or sauce, cream or custard to make foods moist.

Other Useful Tips

1. If you are likely to have a long wait, on a journey, or visit to the clinic, take a nourishing drink or small snack. Even a candy in your pocket will do.

2. Chop your food into bite-sized pieces to make eating easier.

3. Eat your main meal as per the time convenient to you.
4. Eat your favorite foods.
5. Choose fluids that provide some energy – milk, juice, soup etc.
6. Eat and drink slowly.
7. Chew food well. Relax before meals. Anxiety affects the appetite.
8. Rest after eating.
9. Eat with family or friends; eat while watching TV or eat while reading. Your appetite will improve between the treatment. Eat well while you can.

□

Eating is not merely a material pleasure. Eating well gives a spectacular joy to life and contributes immensely to goodwill and happy companionship. It is of great importance to the morale.

—Elsa Schiaparelli

Chapter 10

Prepare Your Own Bucket List

> *"And in the end it's not the years in your life that count. It's life in your years."*
>
> **—Abraham Lincoln**

"Ma'am, are you free on the 2nd of this month" asked Martin.

"I will have to see. What's the matter?" I asked, anticipating some function at his home.

"It's my photographs; I have an exhibition of photographs coming up".

I asked him ***"Since when did you start clicking pics?"***

"Nobody gives credit to the evils we face, but after facing cancer I realized that this evil deserves some credits to my current success. Ma'am I always wanted to be a photographer but never got a chance. When I started receiving chemotherapy I actually found some time to live my childhood dream. Now finally I have time and I want to follow my dream.... though the time is limited". With watery eyes he added with a pause. ***"But I won't have the regret of not chasing my dream before I kick the bucket"***

After Martin left, I had to take a moment to regain myself. The concise conversation was worth a million words.

Life has always been a busy road for us to travel. Even when we were little kids, we could not live our dreams as we were busy matching the expectations of our parents and society. We grew up, pursued careers and lost the touch with our dreams. Our own small cloud of dream was overshadowed by the nimbus of successive responsibilities. And when the time came for the inner kid to reclaim his own life, the disaster 'cancer' struck like lightening. Just imagine all those crazy and weird things you once wanted to do but could not.

□

Make a list of everything you ever wished in your life and couldn't accomplish.

1. **Stay connected to music:** If you are fond of music and ever wished to learn how to play guitar or wanted to learn classical, then there can't be any better time than this. This will keep you busy and also might give you a goal to accomplish. The ecstasy will be unparalleled when you accomplish it.
2. **Globetrotting:** Make a list of places you wanted to visit but couldn't. Plan the trips with family or friends.
3. **Photography:** Grab a camera and start clicking pictures. This may be again a very good hobby to keep you busy.

There are several of such things that you might have thought of doing but couldn't do because of rollercoaster life.

So what are you waiting for, grab a pen and jot down your own bucket list!

My Bucket List

1. ....
2. ....
3. ....
4. ....
5. ....
6. ....
7. ....
8. ....
9. ....
10. ....

> *"Look at the sparrows; they do not know what they will do in the next moment. Let us literally live from moment to moment."*
>
> **—Mahatma Gandhi**

Chapter 11

Life after Cancer – Putting Back the Pieces Together

"I have to get my life back on track. Order as an antidote to chaos. Calm after the storm."

—Susane Colasanti

"It was ironical that in the face of death, I began for the first time, to really live."

—Anup Kumar

Those who have never been through the sufferings, do not know the joy of being a survivor. Our ignorant strata of society has been seen quoting that once you are diagnosed with cancer, even if you complete the treatment; your life will never be the same again. I remember Mr Shadab who once told me that "Though I have completed my treatment and am disease free for years, I still feel that there is always a sword hanging above my head." I could sense the despair in his voice, though he tried to laugh.

A lot of disruption might have occurred during treatment. Studies of children might have been affected. Jobs might have been affected. Financial equations would have changed. But remember one thing – "Things will improve. **Just put the pieces together".**

How each cancer survivor copes with the life after – is very different. It depends a lot on the lessons you learnt during this journey – the journey of cancer. Some emerge stronger than ever. Some continue to live under the fear of recurrence.

One often makes friends with other cancer patients. There will be few who survive and there will be few who are not so lucky. Remember every cancer patient is different. Every person has a different stage and responds in a different manner. Don't feel guilty if someone you knew succumbed to the disease. Neither be grasped by fear. Accept the fact every cancer patient may not have the same journey. Your fate may be entirely different.

Don't let them discriminate against you, because of cancer. People have fought back and won marathons even after the disease. You have emerged stronger than even before, because you have confronted your worst fear. All great men were ordinary men who were forced by circumstances to meet great challenges.

Tips for life – after Cancer:

1. **Be regular** on your follow-ups. Mark your calendar. Set-up alerts about your follow-up visits.

2. Follow **healthy diet** and exercise regularly.

3. **Celebrate** the little moments of triumph and happiness.

4. **Meditate** – it calms mind.

5. **Seek psychologist's help**, if the fear of recurrence predominates your thoughts.

6. **Have a purpose in life**. We were not born only to die. But we were born with a purpose – purpose of being useful. After all, the only other choice is to be useless or used-less.

Remember "*service to humanity is the rent we pay for living on this planet"-Mahatria Ra.* What we do for ourselves, will die with us. What we do for others, will be our legacy.

□

Chapter 12

You are Special

> *"Don't ever doubt yourself or waste a second of your life. It's too short, and you're too special."*
>
> **—Ariana Grande**

You may not realize your own worth but you may mean the entire world for somebody. When we were born, our mothers always held us close to them as their most precious possession. Our first smile, first word we spoke, first steps, just everything was special. And for our loved ones no matter what we do, we will always be special! All it takes is a moment of realization what we mean to others. I have seen patients not valuing their lives.

A young girl named Upasna came for a check-up. I noticed scars on her fore-arm which looked like self-inflicted cuts. When I asked her what are these, she said ***"Mam, I tried to hurt myself because I was upset"!*** I was taken aback how she was so much unmoved by her own acts, as if it was insignificant. I asked her what did your parents feel about it? Her head drooped down in shame! This is not just one patient I came across. I gave her examples of patients who are battling for their lives and so desperately clinging on to every hope to breathe few more breaths. I have seen fathers, mothers, sisters, brothers and wives crying and begging for the cure of their kin.

If you think that you are not special, just peep in the eyes of your loved ones and realize how special you are to them. If you ever feel weak, find your strength in them. If you are sad, find your happiness in your loved ones. Life can never be a bed of roses but one can be thankful for the bed at least. Be thankful for the support you get from your family and relatives.

Life will give you 10 reasons to be sad and might give only one reason to be happy. But that one reason may be worth enough. Moments of joy might be small and sadness may last longer. All of us have a tendency of holding on to the bad memories and we don't even remember the good ones. Take time to think... You are precious. You mean the WORLD to somebody.

□

Chapter 13

Tips for Family, Relatives and Friends

> *"The love of family and the admiration of friends are much more important than wealth and privilege."*
>
> **—Charles Kuralt**

This chapter as the name suggests, is aimed at making friends and family members know their patient better and help him cope up with the treatment. A patient doesn't need your pity. He needs your love and support. A sufferer undergoes so much of transformation that he finds it difficult to cope up with his altered emotional and physical status.

I personally feel that it is equally or probably more difficult for the family members to see the kin in ailment. It was Mr Sukesh who was undergoing treatment for cancer but it was Rajeshwari, his wife who looked more of a patient. Giving care and support to a cancer patient can be challenging at times and may turn out to be frustrating too.

For Family Members

1. Be Sympathetic but don't overdo it

Your constant sympathy and kindness can make the patient nervous. It can also make him wonder whether he is going to die or if there is something about his medical condition that you are not telling him. Spare the patient from the **'pity syndrome'**. Don't remind the patient over and over again that he is not well. Cutting down his physical activity altogether, will make him more depressed.

2. Help him to be independent

The family should realize that the patient is going through the treatment and he may not be able to carry on all those activities, he was doing earlier. It is important to provide him help but **"help him to help himself"**. Maintaining the right balance is important. The patient should not over-exert himself/herself but at the same time he should not be made to feel dependent also. **Remember what the patient needs is not consolation but the motivation to move on.**

3. Listen to him, if he wants to talk

Don't shut him up or change the subject thinking you are doing him good, while not allowing him to talk about his illness. If he wants to talk about his illness, let him talk. Maintaining **'right balance'** is important. Do not always just talk about the disease and illness. Do talk about other things also, to impress upon him that life goes on and he has to fight back. It would be nice to talk about music, movies etc. A break from the 'cancer world' will do him good.

4. Don't cut him off, assuming that he won't to be able to cope up

Maintaining near normal life style within the family unit is extremely important for the self-esteem of the patient. Don't rob him of his role in the family. Let him still maintain the role, whatever he was doing earlier. Just provide help to make things easier. If he was a decision-maker, then let him still be involved with all the decisions of the family. It is important for his self-esteem.

5. Be more tolerant

The patient is bound to suffer from mood swings. There will be depressing moments. Just keep reminding yourself and the patient **"This Too Shall Pass"**.

6. Don't forget to praise him often

The patient is fighting his/her own war of **'body image changes'**. Don't pass harsh remarks. Remember that your relationships may change temporarily but be a little more sensitive. A strong relationship will definitely survive this testing time.

7. Don't be negative

The patient is fighting his own depression. Try to be as positive, as far as possible. A positive atmosphere helps greatly in recovery.

8. Give special attention to diet

Healthy diet is important for everybody but it is all the more important when there is a patient in the family. There can be restrictions in the diet when the person is going through chemotherapy or any other treatment. These restrictions should be discussed in detail with the doctor and notes should be taken. Take care to pass on the instructions clearly to whosoever is preparing the food for the patient, whether it is patient himself/ herself or somebody else.

9. Don't confine him to the boundaries of the house

Many times the family members fear that taking the patient out will exert him or make him susceptible to infections. The patient is often confined to the house or worse, to his room for fear of catching infections. What is important to remember is that patient also needs to live, enjoy life, go out. Do take him out for short trips – may be a car ride. Do take them out for shopping – just avoid the crowded outdoor bazaars. Going to air conditioned spacious malls at non-rush hours and weekdays may be a good idea.

10. Maintain cleanliness

Special attention should be given to the cleanliness of the house. Clean houses invite positive vibrant energy and also give germ-free environment.

11. Make a list of do's and don'ts

Talk in length with your doctor and prepare this list. Keep it at a prominent place where you can see and easily follow the instructions. □

Relatives and friends rush to meet the patient soon after he/she is diagnosed with cancer. And the most disturbing fact about their visit is that they make it look like a 'visit for condolence'. The sufferer imbibes the feeling that he is suffering from incurable disease and is going to die, which is not true in all the cases. They go to meet him using a mask to cover their face fearing they too might get cancer. Understand that he does not want your pity and he is not dying, too. Distant relatives come to the house and cry and start their emotional drama in front of the sufferer. Some relatives do it for 'attendance' purpose. Be sensible, your actions can make things far more worse for others.

For Distant Relatives:

1. **Be constructive than being destructive:** Before you visit the patient, get to know about his emotional status whether he really wants to meet anybody or not. Overdoing things are worse than not doing at all. When you meet him/her, don't act as if it is a condolence visit, don't discuss about the disease even if you know a lot. Discuss about all the positives in life like the relatives, kids, grandchildren and all the things which person loves. Make plans for outings, small trips etc.

2. **Share responsibilities if you can:** Help them find the suitable doctor and hospital regarding the 2nd opinion as and when required.

For friends:

1. **Be the second family:** Friends are considered to be the second family for reasons known to all of us. Make a habit of communicating with your friend because he needs you. Re-live those funny moments again to make your friend forget the agonizing time period.
2. **Be the Shoulder:** Even after completing the treatment, rehabilitation can be a difficult task for a patient. Some are left with physical disfigurement whereas others are low on self-esteem. Help them regain the confidence and strength to walk again. You can be the healing balm for your friend if not physically then emotionally.
3. **Do not disappear:** Always be there for your friend because he needs you at this moment, more than ever. He might not be able to cry in front of his family, but may need you to just let it out. Find out what his needs are, find out appropriate places to hangout, and help him find the shops for wigs, be the fun and above all, be dependable and available.

Warriors' Tales! Stories of Ordinary People...Turned Heroes

Warrior - 1

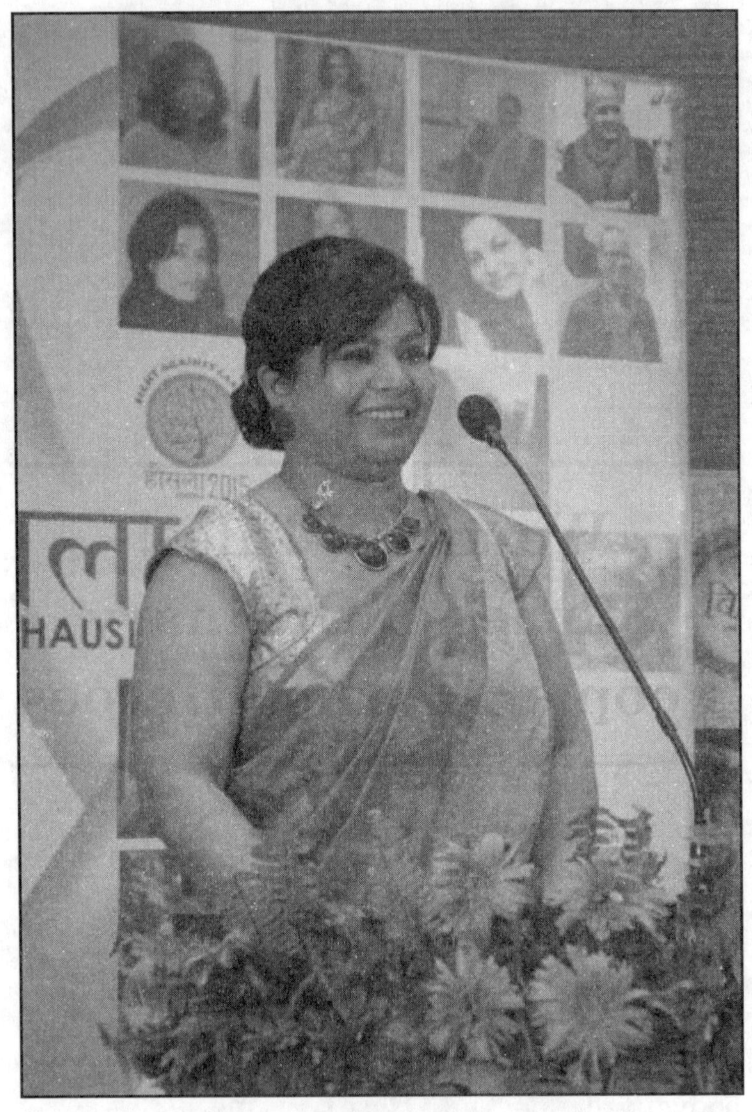

Mrs. Sneha Routray
Diagnosed – 2014
Occupation – Architect

During 2014, it was a great moment for our family when I had gone with my husband and daughter, to see beautiful flora and fauna of beautiful countries like Mauritius and Madagaskar. Like a loving and charming family we enjoyed the trip. Once we got back home, within a few days I felt a lump on my right upper breast. I took it very casually as if nothing serious had happened and that it would subside soon. But then reluctantly, I shared the same with my husband after a while. He was the one who always believe and take early and speedy action for any kind of medical issues. My husband had the privilege to work in Ministry of Health and Family Welfare, Govt of India. Hence, he had the information about such kind of abnormal growth of tissues and so we went for the initial check-up.

My name is Sneha Routray. As directed by our doctor, we immediately went for a biopsy test on the 24th of June 2014. We awaited anxiously but patiently. And when the report arrived, it was a positive. It was reported that I am suffering from breast cancer. My heart dropped. It was totally unacceptable for me since I was fit as a fiddle and there were no symptoms of any sickness just days before. We both were in back seat and our bodyguard along with the driver in the front seat of our car. All of us were at a complete loss of words. At that point of time, both of us were shell-shocked. We sat speechless through the entire journey back home. Although there were so many things to discuss, but for the first time we felt like we needed to hide something from our ever transparent social lives. We just held each others' hands and cried silently. The moment just seemed timeless. We just did not want to discuss about this diagnosis with anyone, specific or in particular. A drooping mélange of anxiety, fear and the future had struck our lives hard, all at the same time. These were our testing times.

After several nervous discussions we immediately went off to Mumbai for surgery. The surgery took place on the 3rd of July at Soumaya Ayurvihar by a senior oncologist. Before the surgery, we went to Sai Baba temple and with a heavy heart I prayed for a peaceful and healthy life ahead or else to grant me a peaceful death during the operation itself. My state of mind was in complete delirium. While entering inside the operation theatre I was really, really scared and simultaneously a myriad of thoughts, of all kinds, were coming to my mind. I forgave everyone who had tried to hurt me; I confessed to God for every single mistake I had made. I thought I was going to die. Scores of faces I knew, through my lifetime were flashing across my eyes. I remembered my grandfather and grandmother's faces.

And the time arrived. The operation took place

for 5 long hours and the deadly lump was finally removed successfully. Though it was difficult for me we felt very relaxed after removal of the lump. It was ductal carcinoma. To our extreme relief, it was initial stage. The same has been sent for test to check whether it was invasive or not. My entire family including my brother, sister, parents, parents-in-law, brother-in-law became the by-standing source of strength for me. All of us were still in tension because on the basis on the reports, chemo and radiation schedule was yet to be decided. I was not prepared and rather too scared for chemo because till that time I had read many articles and was well aware of it being a very painful activity. Finally we got the report and my doctor advised me to go for chemotherapy and target therapy. He referred me to a very senior oncologist whose counseling worked wonders for me. I saw many videos of Yuvraj Singh on Youtube, read several articles on cancer. The more knowledge I gained, the less fear I felt to fight against cancer.

That time, my sweet and lovely daughter, Kinjal was just 5 years old. She was so disturbed with all this in background that her studies were getting affected to no end. Her parents were not with her during those days. I am lucky to have such a wonderful child as Kinjal because despite being totally unaware of what exactly cancer was, she could sense something wrong had happened to my mother. Chemotherapy was conducted successfully, as my parents and my doctor were always there for me. I also overcame the side effects of chemotherapy. Then we all realized early detection of cancer can cure and life span also increases. I actually got a second life. I found many changes within myself in a good way. My inner soul is much beautiful than never before.

You know, cancer changes your life, and oftens for the better. What cancer does is, it forces you to focus, to prioritize, and you learn what's important. I mean, I don't sweat the small stuff. I used to get angry at cab drivers. It's not worth it.... And when somebody says you have cancer, you realize it's all small stuff. And what i say is, if it weren't for the downside, everyone would want to have it. But there is a downside. Then I came in touch with Dr. Meenu Walia under whom my treatment was started. Since then I owe my life to her.

During chemo, you're more tired than you've ever been. It's like a cloud passing over the sun, and suddenly you're out. You don't know how you'll answer the door when your groceries are delivered. But you also find that you're stronger than you've ever been. You're clear. Your mortality is at optimal distance, not up so close that it obscures everything else, but close enough to give you depth of perception.

All shaken but now determined, our organization Grameen Sneh Foundation was determined to have cancer awareness about cancer related issues. In 2009, the GRAMEEN SNEH FOUNDATION had launched the HEALTH, EDUCATION AND SOCIAL related Programme in different activities such as Health, Education early childhood education reform initiative in three states viz. Bihar, Orissa and Delhi-NCR in India. Seven years later, Foundation has developed into a network of individuals working to improve the lives of young children and families through a vibrant learning community active in national and states reform projects. Now the organization has been working in three states New Delhi, Orissa and Bihar in India.The organization is going to move in all over India to make the healthy and disease free India.

Grameen sneh foundation's cancer awareness programme is dedicated to all cancer patients in India, to create a series of awareness regarding feeling of self care and palliative care for the protection and maintenance of healthy and disease-free journey of life. Let's get together instigate and promote – a whole new – fangled sensational wave of awareness, regarding prevention and better cure of cancer by making our beloved ones more aware and conscious about this dreadful, bit curable disease. Our small effort can save someone's precious life. So friends, let's try and create a beautiful cancer awareness programme to fight against cancer.

Now I want to spread this message to

everybody. When I ask myself why me, I get the answer it can happen with anybody and that it completely depends on the lifestyle we maintain. We just can take as an accident. Sometimes when I ask god why he gave me such disease the answer I get is to get into the next level of life. What is next level then?

Next level is, when I conduct cancer awareness programmes and health checkup camps in rural areas of Bihar. Sometimes more than 3000 people come to get screened. A team of 25 to 30 people including doctors and volunteers help in conducting such camps. In every camp we get 6 to 8 cancer detections. We try our level best to facilitate treatment for them. We found many women who were suffering from 3rd stage of cancer and were not even aware of it. Supporting them in some way makes me proud. The happiness I get by doing this can't be described in words. That actually is the next level of life for me.

I met Late Dr. APJ Abdul Kalam sir once to invite him for a cancer awareness programme, which was to be held on 10th of October 2015. Unfortunately he left all of us. He blessed me by saying "EVERYBODY HAS PROBLEM IN DIFFERENT WAYS. THAT MAY BE FINANCIALLY, SOCIALLY OR PHYSICALLY. DEFEAT THE PROBLEM AND CONQUER. EVERYBODY WANTS TO TAKE, THAT'S WHY THE WHOLE WORLD IS SUFFERING.YOU

ARE GIVING TO SOCIETY SO YOU ARE HAPPIEST PERSON.GOD IS WITH YOU THEN WHO CAN BE AGAINST. MY BLESSINGS WITH YOU" (8th June 2015). This was the most proud moment of my life. I am doing all these from my inner soul and will keep on serving the society till the end of my life. Doing such things heal my body and soul. I serve people and this is the path I have chosen to defeat cancer. So in a way, I can say that I was actually blessed by God with cancer. It made me a better person with a brighter and broader perspective. Now I take better care of myself and maintain a healthy lifestyle. Realizing that I am the backbone of my family, I have decided to make myself stronger than ever.

So all my friends, please be strong, be brave like me and tell yourself that cancer is a curable disease. I know this disease gives a lot of pain and life changing negative thoughts but I faced this problem bravely which led to my life changing attitude and emotional feelings for sensibility about humanity for the rest of my life ahead.

So, as a cancer model, I firmly believe that we can make our ways through any difficult ropeway by means of imparting happiness to life and to society.

Sneha Routray

Warrior - 2

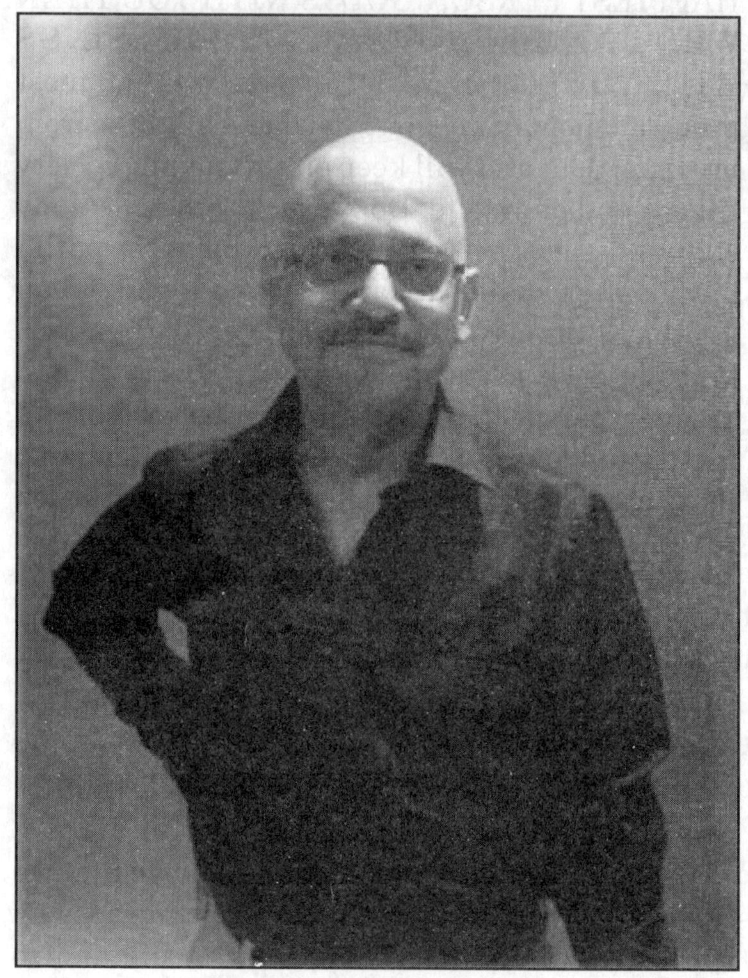

Mr. Pramod Goel
Diagnosed – 2005
Occupation – Business

Hi dear friends,

Today I will share with you some critical moments of my life. I, Pramod Goel, aged 61, a Mechanical Engineer by qualification having served Godrej and Boyce for 23 years in capacity from Executive to Regional Manager. I started my entrepreneurial career with jewellery business in 2003 by the branded showroom of Laabh Jewellers.

The most surprising incident started in 2005 when in a routine health check up at Apollo Hospital, I was suspected diagnosis of cancer in abdomen. I see myself and my small son standing in front of Oncology department, shocked and amazed. We could not believe the diagnosis of the hospital and thought it was a joke. I consulted all the near and dear ones for advice. We went to different hospitals such as Rockland, Rajiv Gandhi Cancer Institute and Dharamshila Hospital for the expert advice.

Finally came in touch with Dr. Meenu Walia at Dharamshila Hospital who very sympathetically and systematically explained the further diagnosis and treatment if required. Within 10 days it got confirmed that Yes,...I was suffering from Cancer, Non Hodgkin's lymphoma in abdomen.

Life was very painful and came to a standstill. Family got utterly depressed. However my wife has a lot of courage to face the challenges ahead. My doctor, Meenu Walia gave us the strength while starting the treatment.

As you all know, treatment of cancer is very tough; money-wise and time-wise. I faced the different phases of treatment with pain and courage. Anyhow, never gave up. Thankful to all the blessings of my family members, near and dear ones, and doctors at Dharamshila Hospital for their unconditional support.

The treatment got completed in 10 months and I was declared fit and free from disease, however I was physically very weak.

Now in 2015, the whole episode looks like a bad dream and I am enjoying my social and family life as usual. As an individual, I suggest and recommend all Cancer patients to fight this disease with a proper treatment and follow up as recommended by the doctors.

I will always be grateful to my doctor and friend Meenu Walia for the treatment imparted and unconditional support during and after the treatment. I am lucky to have her as my doctor.

Many thanks to her!!

Best Regards

Pramod Goel

Warrior - 3

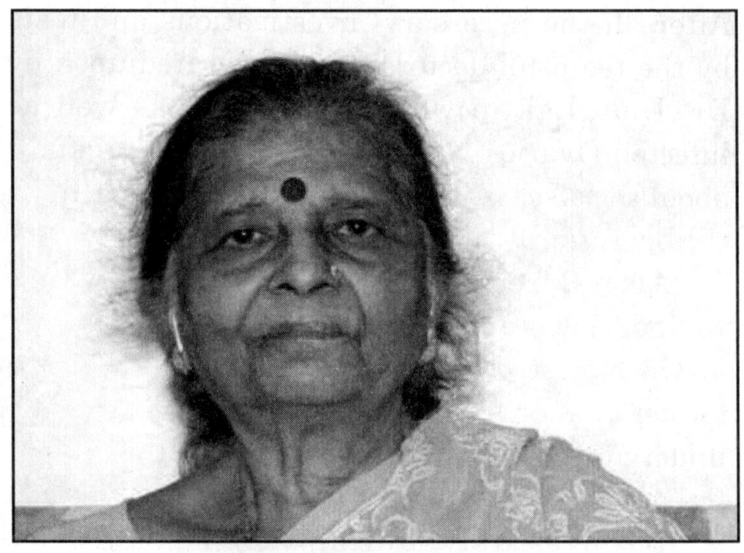

Mrs. Usha Narayan
Diagnosed – 2006

Yes CANCER is curable.

I, Usha Narayan, aged 76 years, previously a patient of dreaded disease is now completely cured.

In the month of July 2006, I was diagnosed as a patient of Cancer. This fact was closely guarded secret by my two sons till it was operated upon. After all the necessary investigations and tests by the teams of doctors, I was operated upon by Dr. Uma Rai. in which my Uterus as well as infected Ovaries were removed. I came to know about the disease in the ICCU of the hospital after the operation.

After I recuperated from the procedure wounds, I was advised to seek further advice from an Oncologist. We consulted Dr. MEENU WALIA for her opinion and treatment. She advised me to undergo CHEMOTHERAPY which, I took under the precise treatment of Dr. MEENU WALIA.

Unfortunately, during the chemotherapy treatment, within a year, I, suffered fracture of my vertebral column. Again marathon of treatment for fractured vertebral column started along with Chemotherapy, which in due course, I recovered. After the completion of Chemotherapy within couples of months, I, was again operated upon for hernia.

During this difficult phase of my life my Husband, my Daughter and my two Sons and their respective families helped me a lot and boosted my morale. They never treated me as a cancer patient but they insisted me to believe me that "I WAS DISEASE FREE NORMAL PERSON AS THEY WERE". First I could not believe them but thereafter by God's Grace, I was able to shed my fear and taboo regarding cancer. I made my WILL POWER strong to fight against the cancer. With the support of my family members, I was able to overcome my pain and kept smiling and made myself active.

During the entire treatment of Chemotherapy, I walked into the hospital myself and never subjected myself to the mercy of wheel chair. I still do all my domestic chores myself as was done by me before the treatment.

I am really grateful to all my doctors Dr. Rajeev Moteini, Family doctor, Dr. Uma Rai, Dr. APS Bedi, and Dr. Meenu Walia who guided and treated me, whom I owe my life.

I won the FIGHT AGAINST THE CANCER by my 'WILL POWER' and 'POSITIVE ATTITUDE' towards life.

Usha Narayan

Warrior - 4

"At any given moment,
YOU have the POWER to say:
This is NOT how the story
is going to END."
~ Christine Mason Miller
BLISS
Beautifying Lives, Strengthening Souls

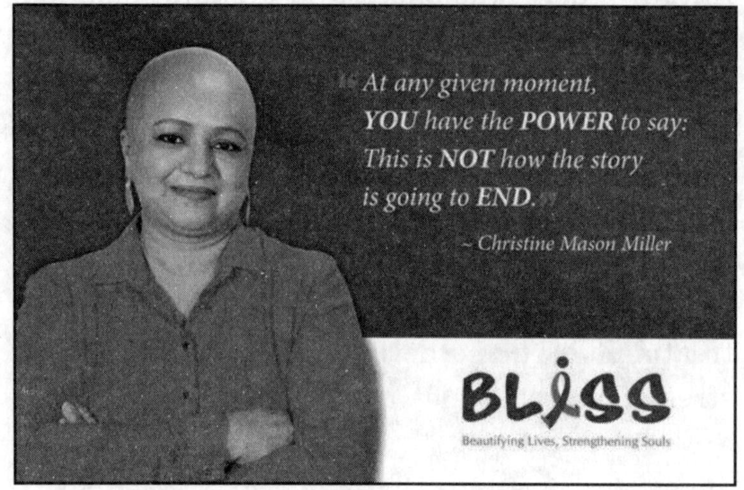

Mrs. Nidhi Agarwal

Diagnosed – 2014

BLISS: 'Beautifying Lives Strengthening Souls' is the brainchild of me and my son Aayush Agarwal.

My cancer was found completely by chance in 2014. Like many others, I had no signs or symptoms. I self-detected myself and was diagnosed with breast cancer – just like that. Initially there was shock and dreadful emotion, but it soon gave way to action. I did not dwell on the fact that I had cancer – I knew I had to act fast and do all that is needed to beat the disease. Within a week of being diagnosed, I had a mastectomy and reconstructive surgery. I battled a lot of pain but remained positive and resilient all along. Then began the painful and agonising treatment of chemotherapy. The treatments were stressful both physically and emotionally for me and my family. The changes in physical appearances, intense fatigue and constant pain were just some of the things I learnt to cope with on a daily basis. Hair loss, changes in skin texture, discolouration of nails, weight gain were other fallouts I was faced with. My changing condition prompted reflection and I realised that accepting the disease was the only way to deal with it. I was undergoing my chemotherapy sessions at MAX Hospital. Here I came across the Cancer Support Group at MAX Hospital. It was an inspiration in itself. I was no longer a patient of cancer, rather I was a survivor. I met some of the most inspiring and brilliant doctors such as Dr. Geeta, Dr. Vineeta, Dr. Meenu, Dr. Randeep and made some long lasting friends. The Thursday meetings, those engaging discussions, all the fun activities somehow became a part and parcel of my life and battling the disease was much easier now. At one of the forums for breast cancer patients in Max Hospital I realised what my next purpose was. Being a cancer survivor had made me some kind of celebrity and, in my characteristic confident manner; I found in cancer a style statement of my own. Knowing more about the disease had helped me become more confident about my faith and my ability to help others facing the same trauma. Far from seeing the wreckage of a life, I found the strength to pick up all the threads and start over again. Through repeated hospital visits, I and my son realised that women undergoing cancer treatment descend into dark and deep depression. They lack motivation and the thought of looking good simply disappears. I decided to help them. I started to leverage my experience and knowledge of the cosmetic industry to help and motivate breast cancer survivors to look and feel good. And this was the genesis of 'BLISS'. I am really thankful to my family, friends and most of all the members of the MAX Hospital for helping me through my difficult time. I hope to be successful in my initiative and touch the hearts of many survivors like me.

Thanks with regards

Nidhi Agarwal

Warrior - 5

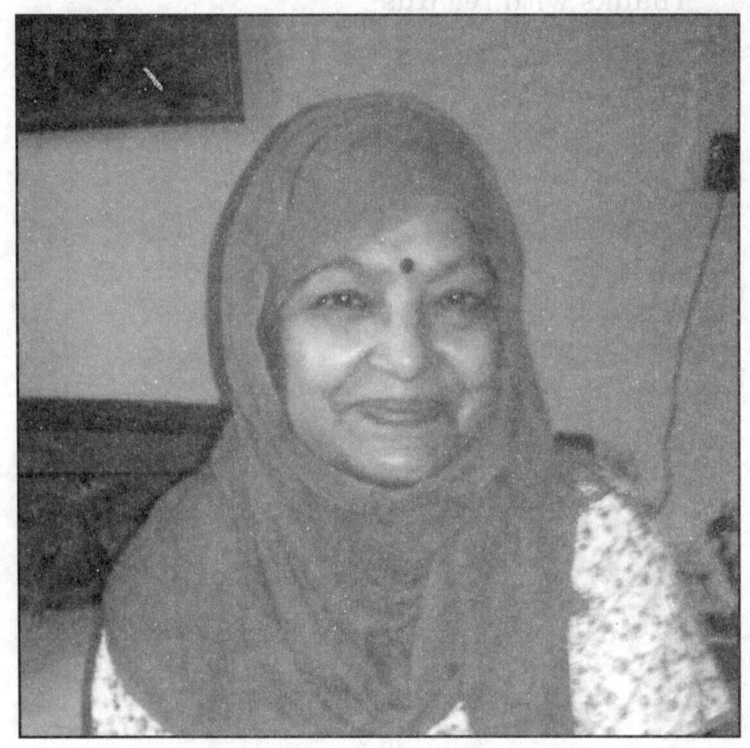

Mrs. Leela Joshi
Diagnosed – 2015

Dawn and Dusk

Just like a day, life has two phases dawn and dusk and it can flip anytime. The way the crack of dawn brings with itself sunshine and fills our life with new hope and zeal, the same way the silence and darkness of the dusk can bring us misery in the form of mental and physical agony.

When I sit and think about all the roles I played in my life and all the memories I made, I get a sense of pride, satisfaction and happiness. From being a pampered and a doting daughter of my parents to being a responsible wife to my husband and a mother-cum-friend to my daughters, I have always tried to fill my family's lives with love and joy. With passing years, new relations were built and I started reliving my childhood with my grandchildren.

Sailing in the boat of my life I didn't realise when cancer in the form of dusk overshadowed the sunshine I was living under. Merely the word Cancer shook my confidence and faith and my world came tumbling down in front of me.

Since December 2014, I was suffering from chronic stomach ache. Suddenly one day in Ahmedabad as I was suffering from unbearable pain I was admitted in the hospital. After a series of tests, I was diagnosed with this deadly disease, endometrial cancer which unfortunately had spread in my abdomen.

As there were better medical facilities in Delhi, my family decided to continue with my treatment in Max Hospital, Delhi which has a reputed oncology department.

From 11th February, 2015 my treatment started under Dr. Meenu Walia. My body negatively responded to the first chemotherapy and I felt that this is where it all ends and its time to say goodbye. But the proactiveness and efficiency of the entire team of doctors and the nursing staff helped me to narrowly escape my end.

So far I have been given 7 cycles of chemotherapy with each cycle comprising of 3 sittings, and the pain and suffering has only made me a stronger person. Now I have come down to medicinal treatment from chemotherapy and I feel better and more hopeful about myself as a patient.

This makes me believe that the advancement of science and technology can make anything possible which is also leading to better life expectancy of patients with diseases like that of mine.

My daughter, Kummu and her family have been at my constant service and Dr. Meenu Walia has left no stone unturned in my treatment. With support like this I feel I'am defeating the darkness of the dusk and the sun is again shining over me.

Thus, I am now a part of the Hausla Group and by participating in their program I wish to inspire and encourage other patients to fight the cancer battle with strength and positivity.

Leela Joshi

Warrior - 6

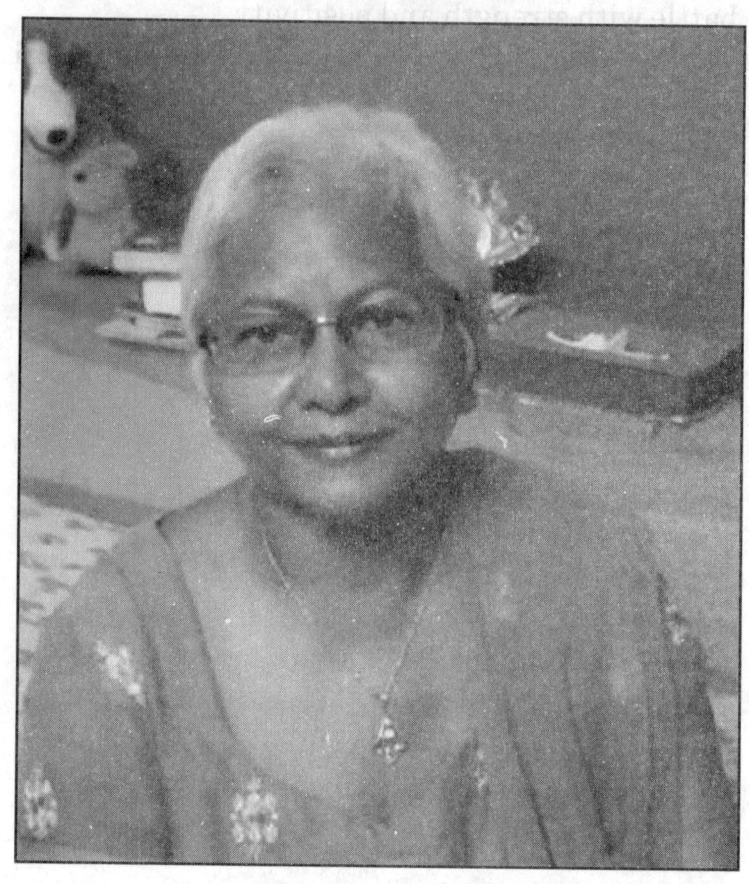

Mrs. Anju Gupta
Diagnosed – January 2015

'Cancer', I have come to view this word as a journey towards self-discovery. My first encounter with cancer was when my mother at the age of 73, was diagnosed with cervical cancer. After a year of harsh medicines, I watched helplessly as she finally surrendered to death. The experience left a tremendous scar in my heart. I feared Cancer. This is probably why when I was first diagnosed with Breast Cancer less than a year ago, I was apprehensive about the treatment. What good would it do for me when none of those medicines could help my mother?

To this day, I thank my stars for finding Dr. Meenu Walia. She was a powerhouse of inspiration and encouragement for me. I particularly remember this conversation with her where she was telling me about the improvement in medicinal science. She told me that my cancer is about 80% curable. I responded, "Why not a 100%?" to which she said "Anju, if today you were to get out of your house you still run a risk of atleast 20% of getting hit by a car. It's not a bad rate of survival." She really did point me in the right direction at whenever that I wanted to turn back. My family, my doctors and my support group have ensured that I walk on this path of self-discovery. Simple things like getting my treatment done, substituting my diet with healthy and natural food, going for regular walks have made me even healthier than I was before. For me survival can be summed up in 3 words – Never Give Up. That's the heart of it really. We just need to keep forging ahead.

Anju Gupta

Warrior - 7

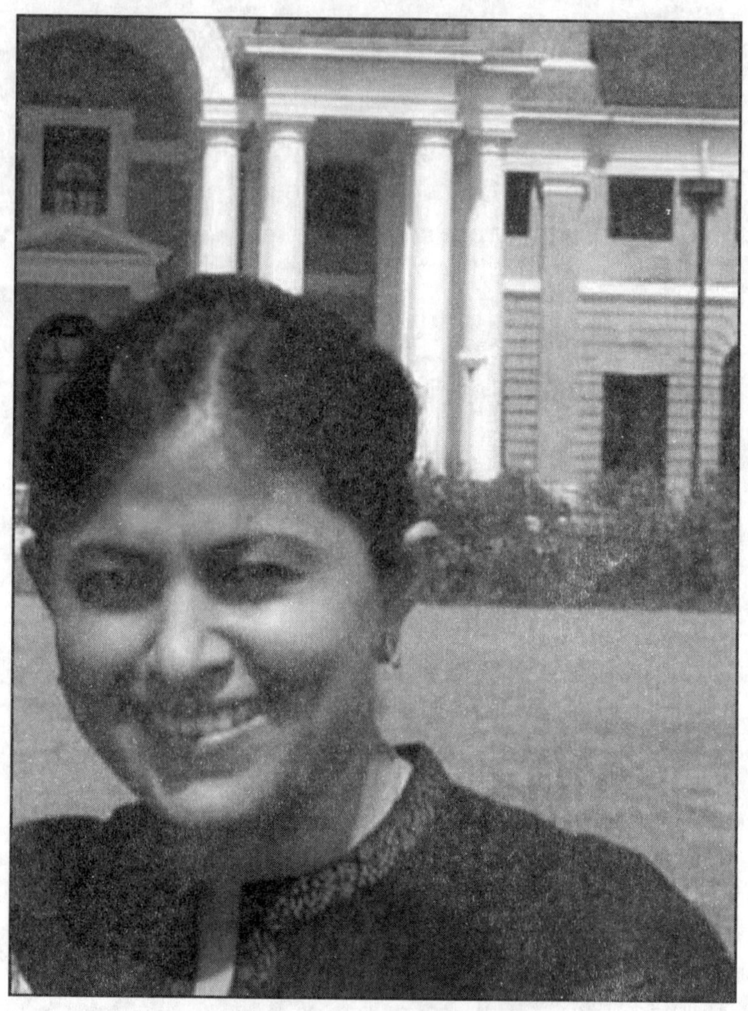

Mrs. Manjusha Shukla
Diagnosed – March 2010

"Live life to the fullest"

Having the disease and living through its cure taught me one thing about life that it is highly unpredictable and we should live it to the fullest with whatever time we have. My strength in recovery was unparalleled family support and faith in doctor.

It is a very difficult phase of life knowing that you have cancer and it becomes more difficult because of the pain enclosed in its cure. There is less public awareness about the disease and the precautions to be taken during the medication.

I hope such events are organized more regularly so that the patients are motivated and get strength to fight the disease seeing the people who have cured and are in remission.

Manjusha Shukla

Warrior - 8

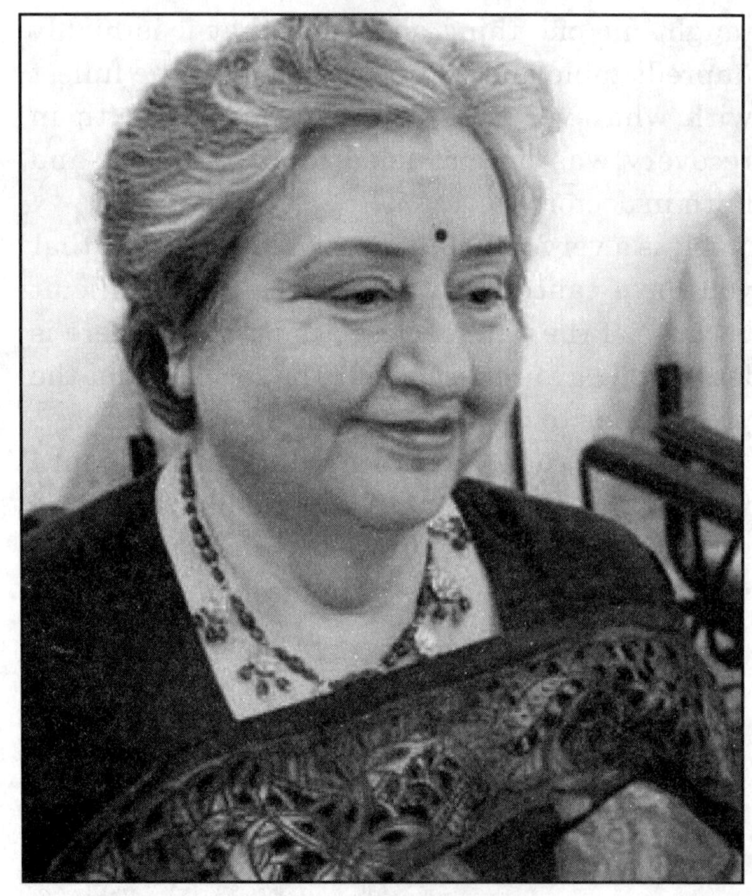

Mrs. Manju Katiyal
Diagnosed – 2014

Mantra: Lets Censor the Cancer!!!

Warrior - 9

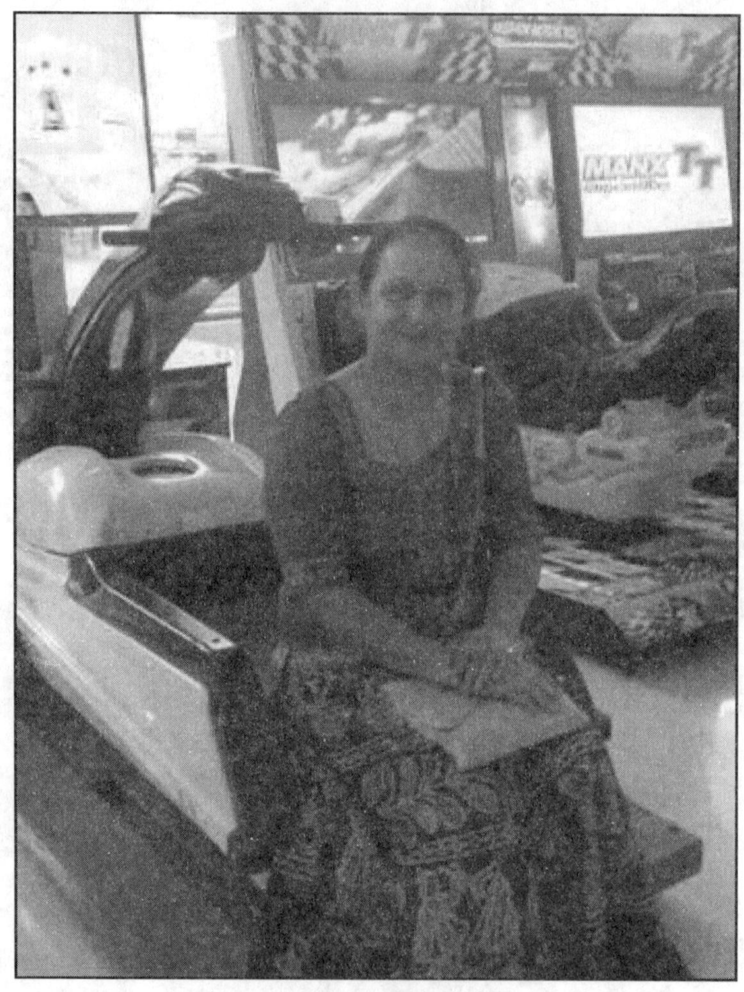

Mrs. Meenu Gulati

Diagnosed – 2013

Cancer is a challenge given to God's
beloved to make them stronger and to become
the inspiration to
others. During the struggle stage, the person
gets broken into pieces
but time cures everything. I was a cancer patient
but I found my life
in my family. It is ultimately your choice either
to be victim or a survivor.

Meenu Gulati

Warrior - 10

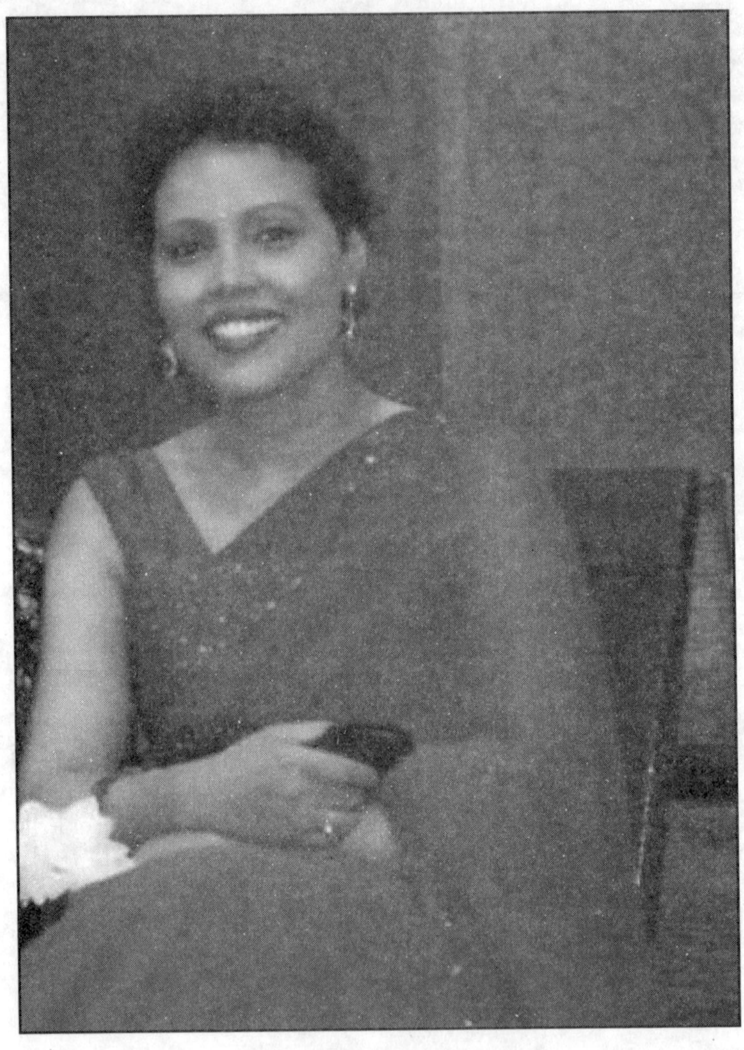

Mrs. Opel Rawat
Diagnosed – 2014

Cancer is not a disease,
its a battle that can be fought with faith
"I WILL WIN". It can take away all of
my abilities but can't touch my mind,
heart and soul, till I keep positive attitude
"I will overcome from it".
We only get one life, live it fully.
Keep smiling

Opel Rawat

Warrior - 11

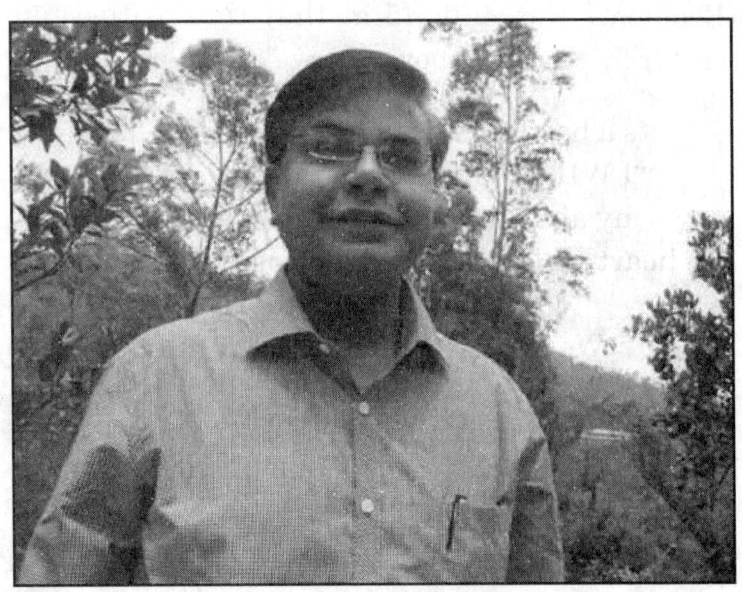

Mr. Irshad Ahmad
Diagnosed – 2014

Since the middle of 2014, I was consistently losing weight and was also keeping mild fever frequently. My General Physician thought diabetes/tuberculosis as the reason behind it. In Feb. 2015, I felt a lump in left side of the neck. CT scan, Biopsy and IHC test diagnosed it as Classical Hodgkin Lymphoma. Initially I was devastated as the name cancer itself is enough to fear about. Besides I was only 45 at that time with small children to care about. However thanks to my doctor Meenu Walia at Max Patparganj and my family, who made me believe that it is fully curable. Although it is a time consuming treatment but after six cycles of chemotherapy, I am feeling quite confident and having this gut feeling that the disease has almost vanished.

Irshad Ahmad

Warrior - 12

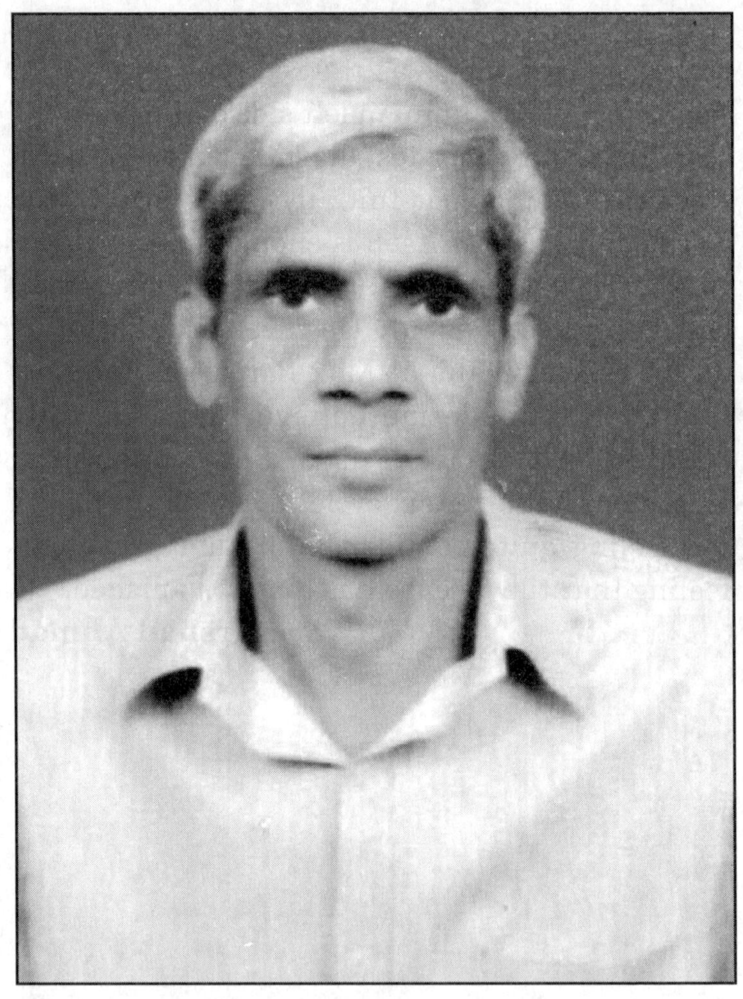

Mr. Basant Kumar Kabra

Diagnosed – 2014

"Cancer can take
away all of my physical abilities. It cannot touch
my mind, it cannot
touch my heart, and it cannot touch my soul"

Basant Kumar Kabra

Warrior - 13

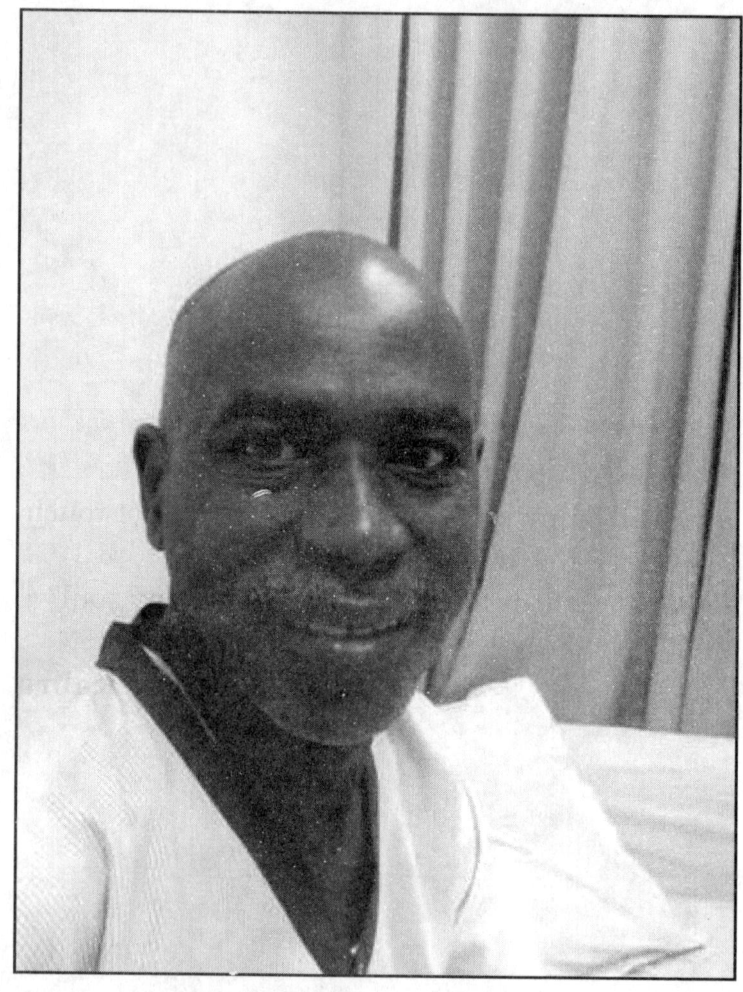

Mr. Ahmad Abdullah
Diagnosed – 2015

"From Sudan to India for the treatment has been full of doubts, new country new people. But as they say that wait till the unrest of water to calm before you can see a clearer reflection of yourself. It takes time with lot of faith and courage. Aren't you brave enough for the one fight?"

Ahmad Abdullah

Warrior - 14

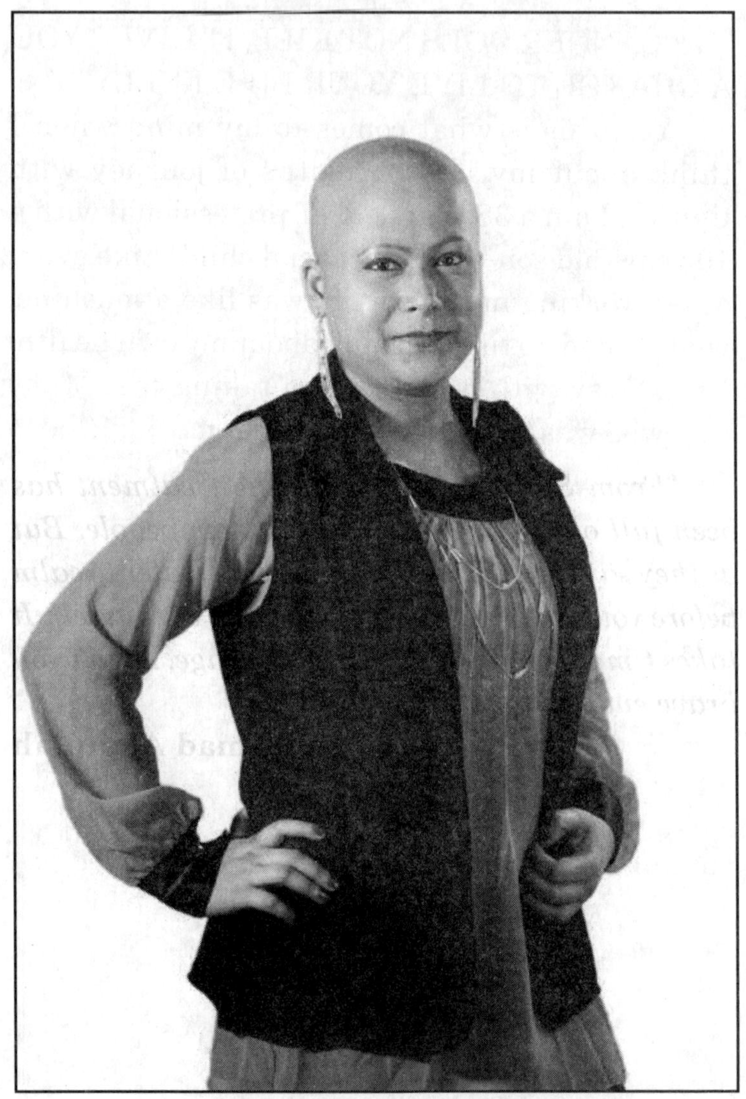

Parimita Sahoo
Diagnosed – 2015

“CANCER DOES NOT KILL, IT GIVES YOU A CHANCE TO LIVE YOUR LIFE FULLY”

Yes, this is what comes to my mind when I think about my last 6 months of journey with Cancer. I am a 38 years old IT professional with a 10 years old son who is a special child. Like every other working mom, my life was like a machine, where I had no time to think about my own health. I was busy with my work and taking care of my son, who was heavily dependent on me. I had been thinking of taking a long break from the hectic schedule when I suddenly found that I have CANCER...a word which I never thought of. I never even googled this word ☺. Honestly, like every other ordinary women, I got devastated as I thought I am dying and I was not ready for that. I had to live for my son, for my family and I wanted to spend quality time with them which I never got. And I think this is what gave me strength and courage to fight against all negative thoughts and I very soon accepted the situation as I got a very good reason to enjoy my cancer, i.e., my much needed long break and lot of time that I could spend with family. I was always very strong, but cancer made me stronger. It did not break me or my family, rather, my son is now very much self-dependent and taking good care of me. It made me so strong that I have been travelling from Odisha to Delhi every week on my own for the chemotherapy leaving my family behind. It gave me a passion to do something for the society. Today I am confident that "Cancer can never kill me" as it had taught me how to live my life fully.

Parimita Sahoo

Warrior - 15

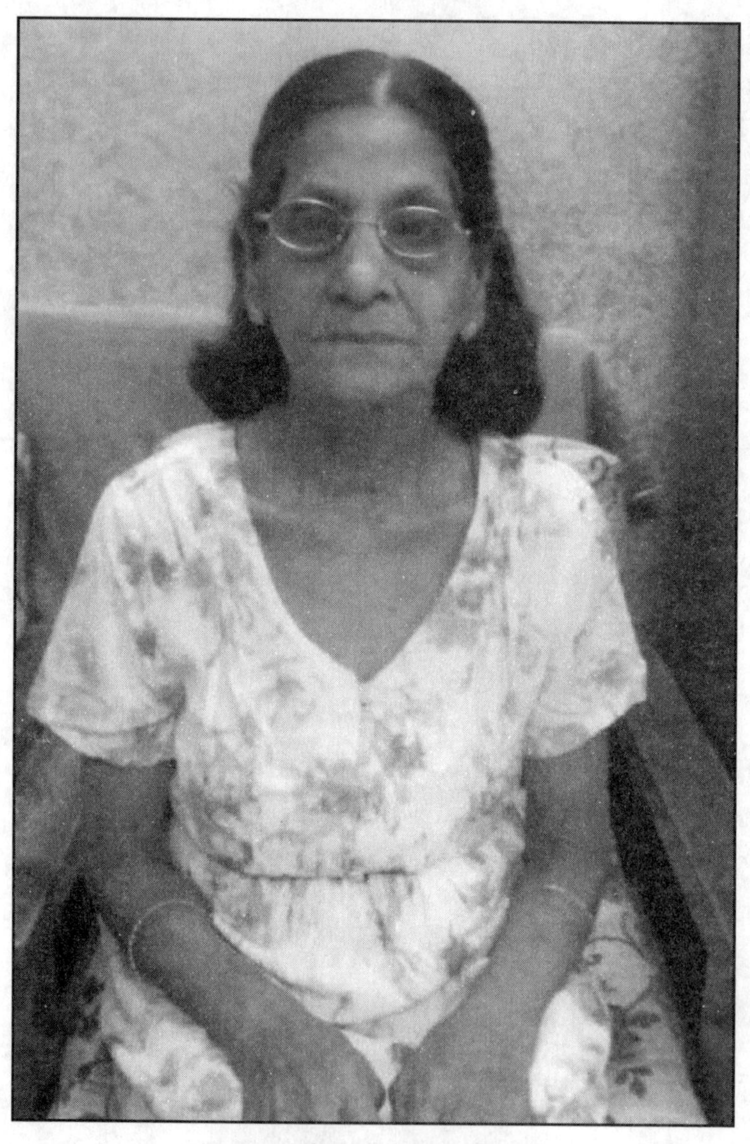

Mrs. Clarita Menezes
Diagnosed – 2009

In the year November 2009, my mother was diagnosed with Lymphoma 3rd stage as informed to me by the person who did the ultrasound. This goes without saying that this information left us all badly shattered, At that moment I did not divulge this news to my mother because she was anyway too weak and has lost a lot of weight and I did not want to alarm her.

All I told her was that she had a lump in her stomach which needed to be dissolved and for which we were to go for a treatment to 'Dharamshila Hospital'.

This she believed and we started her treatment under the Oncologist Dr. Praveen and later Dr. Meenu Walia. With the passage of time and treatment (Chemo) it started to dwell on her that she had cancer as she saw the hair loss and other signs which were a pointer to the disease, but the strong point was that she did not give up She fought the disease with a strong determination and with prayer.

On completing her 12 circles of chemo, we took permission from the Oncologist to take her to "The Divine retreat Centre/Kerala" in the year 2010 where we put her under the care and healing of the greatest Doctor 'our Lord Jesus'. On completing the retreat, which she did most satisfactorily we returned home and went for a check up to Dr. Meenu Walia, who advised us a pet scan, the results of the pet scan were NEGATIVE for cancer and till date my mother has shown no signs of cancer.

Today being 81 years old, she is very active and does all the house work, goes for her walks and of course prayers a lot. The focal point was her strong determination and will power not to give in to the disease and her total surrender in faith to our Lord Jesus.

Ivan Menezes

(Clarita's son)

Warrior - 16

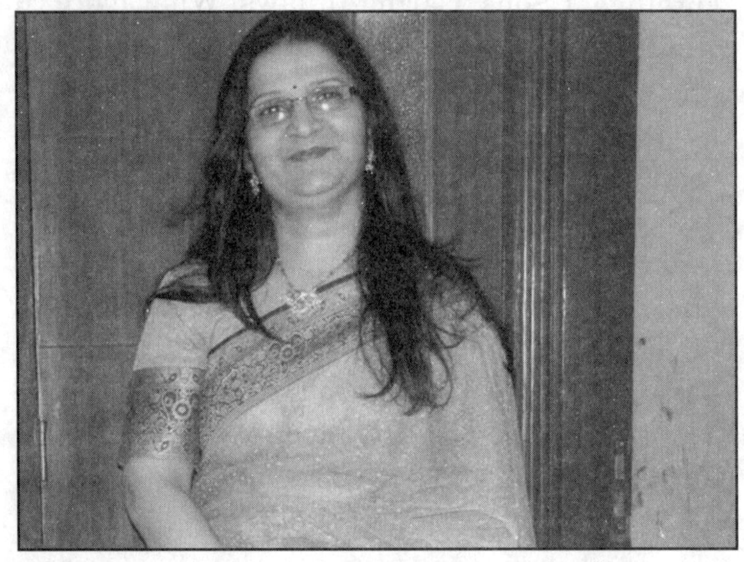

Vandana Anand
Diagnosed – 2015

You never know how strong, you are till the time, being strong is the only option you have.

Above mentioned lines summarise myself and my experience.... Life was going like a fairy tale for me...17 fun filled years of togetherness in married life. A loving husband, 2 smart and intelligent Sons, Caring In-laws. What more can a women ask for in her life? I was like on top of the world.

Before going into the details of my story, I would like to offer my gratitude to all those who have helped me in my battle against this disease... Apart from my family I would sincerely like to thank my doctors from Max Patparganj and their team. Dr. Geeta Kadyaprath for her friendly and bubbly nature and for keeping me motivated. The calm and composed Dr. Meenu Walia for giving me the confidence that I will come out of this ordeal with flying colours and I should not be worried... The lovely ladies and people in Max support group, who were always there to help and give me those important tips during my treatment..

This diagnosis of Breast Cancer turned my life upside down for a while. It was in March-2015 when I first felt a small lump in my left breast. Initially I took it lightly but after about 2-3 days I discussed it with my husband, who told me to go and consult a doctor as he was a bit busy in his financial year end targets. Waited for another 2-3 days and then turned on to my Gynae (a one stop solution for all the females) who asked me to immediately rush for mammography and Ultrasound. Initial findings were somewhat terrifying for me and my husband. We took the reports to our family friend and Doctor (Dr. Paras Gangwal) who asked us to immediately have an appointment with a cancer specialist and get the biopsy done.

I remember it was on March 25th when I entered Max Patparganj, Hospital for the first time and got my Biopsy done there. I was terribly scared and finally when on March 30th my husband got the Biopsy report on his email, he was literally in tears. I rarely saw him reacting like this during 17 years of our togetherness. He is an introvert and never believed in expressing his love but those tears described everything. The next day, when he was getting my Bone Scan done, I saw him shivering and literally praying to god for my well being. That simple question and thought, that why this disease has happened to my wife was disturbing him and somehow this thought disturbed me also.

This pain of my husband somehow made me very strong and that was the day I decided to forget my own pain and to take this disease head on with a very positive frame of mind and approach. I decided that I will bravely overcome all this for my loving family. All the scary thoughts then diminished. The Surgery (Left Mastectomy) was performed on 7th April and in between the period of my surgery and Chemo, I took this task of preparing myself emotionally and mentally strong. I started reading some biographies and motivational articles and while doing this I read a very sweet comment I think from Charlie Chaplin which stated that "Cry as much as you want to, but make sure when you are finished you don't cry for the same reason again". I treated these lines as Geeta Saar in my life. There was no place for tears in my life after this.

Life is a bit tough to get used to after this disease as all the pretty body parts of a lady is affected. We loose one of our important body part, We loose our hair, get cuts and scars. Its really tough for any lady to accept these physical changes BUT I asked myself and want to tell every lady who is going through this treatment that "Are these pretty body parts more important than our family whom we love so much? My husband, family and some of my friends were very supportive and thats what you need during the entire course of your treatment. There should not be any place for negativity and negative thoughts apart from having a good support system around you. Stay away from negative people and start loving yourself. I did the same and this feeling has empowered me. I have started loving myself and now my doctors and friends also compliment me that I look better than before.

So friends! my motivational mantra is that take the disease head on as you can't change what has already happened to you and whats there in your destiny. Identify your support system and stay away from negative people and thoughts. Enjoy your womanhood to the fullest and you will surely succeed...Amen!

Vandana Anand

Warrior - 17

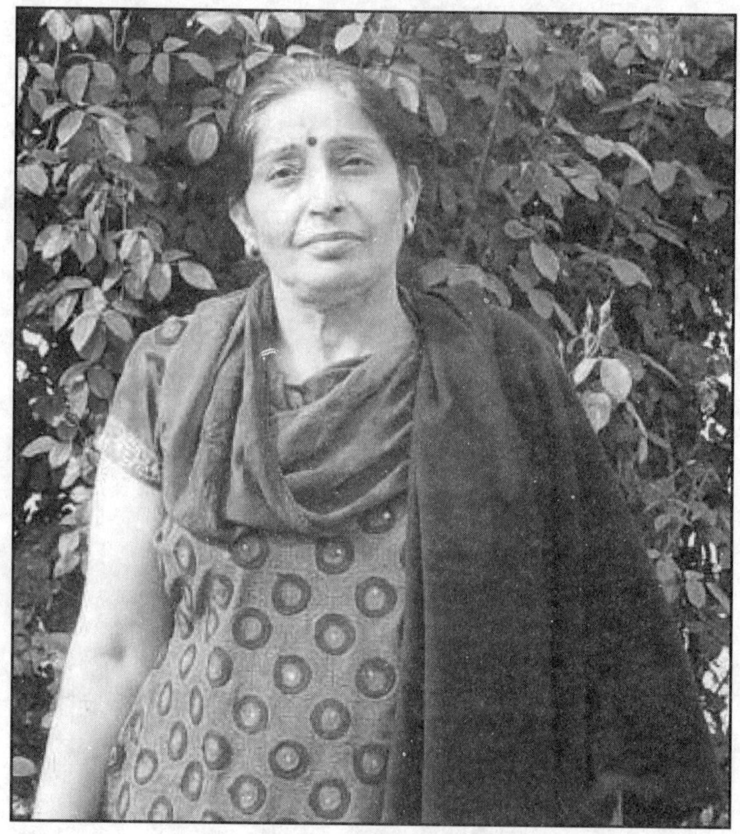

Mrs. Kanchan Malhotra
Diagnosed – March, 2013

wo khud hi tey krte hai manzil aasmano ki
parindo ko nhi di jaati taalim udaano ki
rakhte hai jo hausla aasmaan chhoone ka
unko nhi parwaah kbhi gir jaane ki

Kanchan Malhotra

Warrior - 18

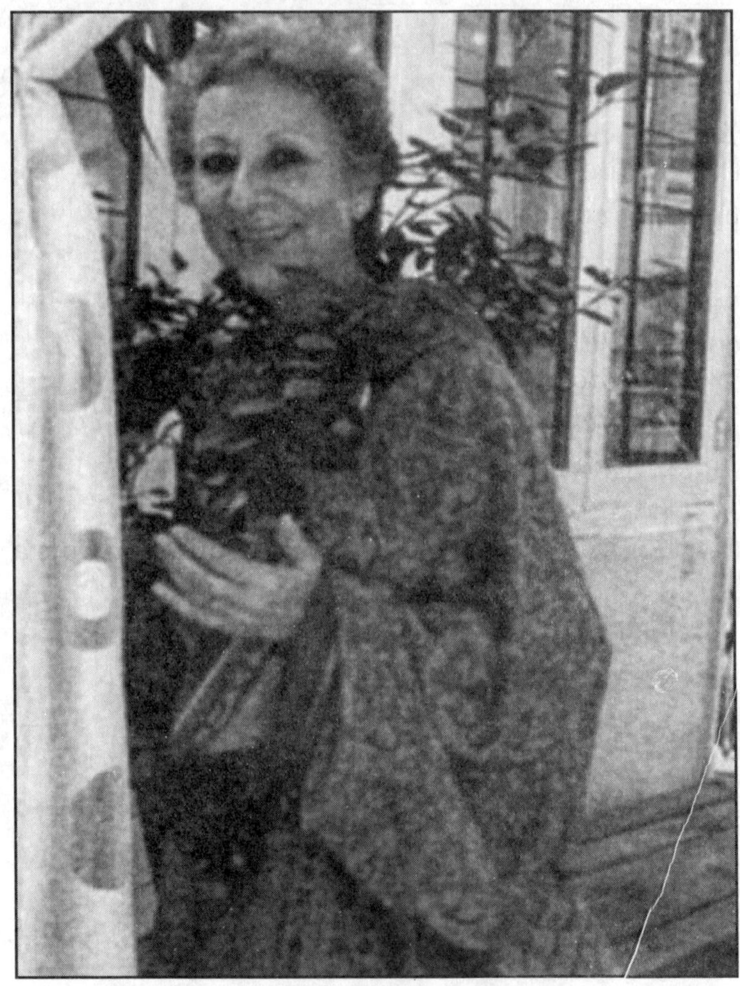

Mrs. Madhu Nanda
Diagnosed – October, 2009

I CHOKED... I CRIED
I BATTLED... I WON

Cancer does not make you unique but it definitely makes you different!

You start living life with a passion enjoying the smallest of things! Life just becomes more precious and everything around more valuable.

A gesture of someone giving you a glass of water or medicine or a home becomes a culmination of love!

My story started with tremendous agonising unbearable pain in the year 2009 when I was diagnosed with B. Cell Lymphoma in my spine. I had to go through an immediate surgery under the distinguished Dr. Bipin Walia at Max Hospital Saket. who came with a magic wand, followed by Radiation under Dr. Anand and his very efficient technical team.

There after I was taken for Chemotherapy to Dharamshila hospital under Dr. Meenu Walia.

My journey had begun....

I was engulfed with pain, tears,defeat, anguish, helplessness and so much had to be done!

Dr. Meenu came like a whiff of fresh breeze. I at once took to her felt comfortable and assured.

My sessions of chemo started and my counts started playing their game. With spells of nausea uneasiness depression and sadness.

I was at my lowest edge.

A sad bad phase....!

Now the best part of the story.

When I was totally low and undermined, I only thought of our Saint. Om Shakti Baba in whom we have complete faith. I bow to Him in complete gratitude and reverence.

My sisters, my children and family stood by me – as tall pillars of strength and motivation. They made me smile laugh cry and helped with just everything. Grand children offered a new hope, a new dawn. They gave me a Home and relaxed breathers with tea/ coffee.

Every fond talk is recorded in the memoirs of my grey matter. I started feeling so blessed that I thanked Him again and again for sending the right people in my life. ...I continued to pray and asking for His constant support.

My family kept saying I had to be back and live again, travel, enjoy, have fun!

These words rang a bell!

I started being more disciplined, exercising. walking and most of all smiling and reading.

A year of unbalanced life followed with a lot of joy. All who trespassed my path contributed either in imparting happiness, or hurting me. I learnt to be brave and courageous, negating the negative and the karma theory. I had to improve my karma.

The process of healing was in progress!

I now live, love, laugh and survive totally because of His Grace. The angels, He has sent in my life in the form of my family and my doctor.

I still have to strive to keep swimming upwards into a life of rejoicing and keep myself afloat.

Eat, Love and Pray.

Life is breathtakingly beautiful!

Enjoy every moment that God gives us.

Madhu Nanda

Warrior - 19

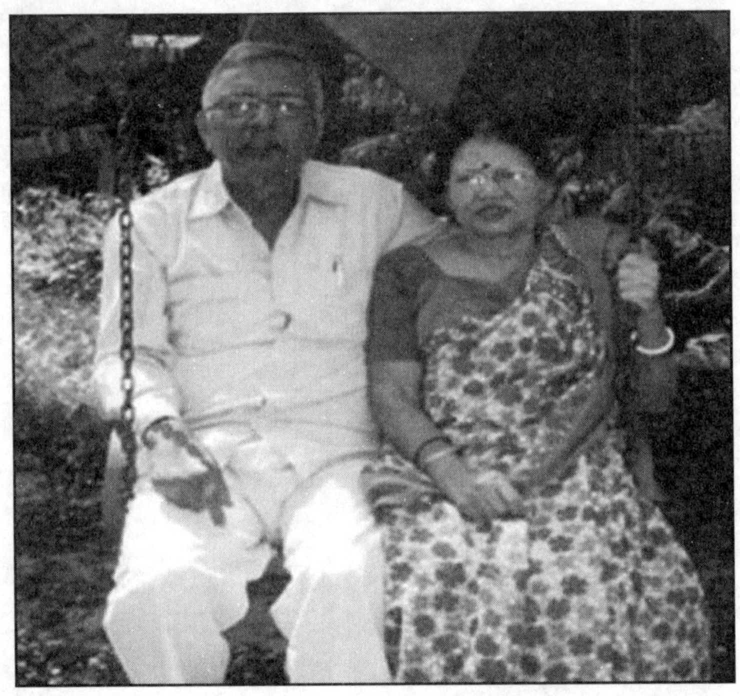

Mrs. Anushila Bhattacharya
Diagnosed – 2014
Mr. Prabuddha Bhattacharya
Diagnosed – 2017

Grandma's philosophy of life was: '*Do what seems like a good idea on time and do it as best as possible.*' It had never let her down and it's still valid today (Dadi *Ma ki nuskhe*).

The same strategy was adopted by my parents: '*Stay low, stay quiet, keep it simple, don't expect too much, and enjoy what you have...*'

Both my parents, Prabuddha Kumar Bhattacharyya and Smt. Anushila Bhattacharya, brilliant in academics, settled in the steel township of Durgapur during the formative days of the eminent city, living life according to the tag line: '*There is a little bit of SAIL in everybody's life.*'

A state gold-medallist, BE/M.Tech. in Operational Research, my father contributed immensely in various departments of SAIL, both in India and abroad. He founded the Panchabati Society, meaning 'Abode of Five Banyan Trees', which is an epitome of togetherness, still residing in the hearts of the steel township.

With Masters in her kitty, my mother chose the teaching profession and excelled as Mathematics Lecturer with a huge fan following amongst the student population – a rare feat in this discipline.

Having groomed three children to their respective successful lives, they are now faced with the demon of modern-age pollution and lifestyle – the dreaded CANCER!!

It was the summer of 2014, just after *Baisakhi,* when Ma came to Delhi from Kolkata and complained about having some projected stomach tissue, which looked like hernia. We consulted our family doctor, who recommended a visit to the Head of the Department of gastroenteritis at Fortis and who, in turn, advised CT scan. The results were horrifying. We were numbed with shock. It was our first encounter with cancer and we did not know what to do, where to go...the world around us just stopped spinning! Ma was diagnosed with ovarian cancer, stage 4.

Baba's case was highlighted during the routine check-up by our family doctor, when PSA results were marginally high and had been consistent for quite long. The first biopsy at a local clinic revealed nothing but the PSA results continued to be the same. So, we went in for the second biopsy at Max Hospital at Patparganj where prostate cancer, stage 2 was detected.

Our first thought was, 'O God! Why this??'

Both Baba and Ma faced this deadly disease stoically. Initially, after receiving the cancer diagnosis, they had been at a loss. The thought of living with cancer and undergo the painful treatment process was extremely overwhelming. We started contacting our relatives, friends, so that they could provide some pointers.

Once the hospital and doctors had been decided

upon, the next course of action began and became fast paced. Hours turned into days and poured past night; days turned into weeks and so on ... we lost track of time. Everything was controlled invisibly; we felt like puppets in the hands of Fate. At some point during the treatment, Ma felt like giving up hope, but we all hung on.

On the onset, one of the reputed hospitals goofed up her case and she went into coma and ventilator support for straight 16 days...we almost lost her! We contacted five reputed hospitals in NCR and out-station; except for doctors at Max Hospital, all other experts gave four months' time-frame longevity (that was seven years back).

Both have been struggling with this dreadful disease for the past five-and-a-half years now, but they keep on inspiring everyone around them with their energy, zest and liveliness. There is a 'CAN' in the word 'CANCER' and they are determined to beat it...emphasising the statement that 'broken crayons still colour', beautifully.

Ma had to be hospitalised 27 times (for chemotherapy mainly). There were moments of desperation with fear of losing her loomed large in the dark corners of our mind. On one night in ICU, I remember standing hopeless...praying to God...Baba had to undergo months of hospitalisation due to radiation therapy and he bore all the sessions sportingly!

The doctors (Dr. Meenu Walia and team) stood by us like a rock and held our hand, steadily guiding us with innovative treatment interventions, detailed planning and attending to all emergencies with an assuring surety.

The day when Ma got admitted, she was in severe pain and discomfort. She had had a little accident that morning when she had slipped in the bathroom. We admitted her to one hospital, only to transfer her to Max at Patparganj when the situation worsened. By late night, she was admitted to ICU and her condition kept on going downhill from there. Both kidney failure, fluid accumulation in both lungs, cardiac dysfunction, comatose...*it was such a hopeless, dark situation.* I glued myself to the first floor ICU lounge for five straight days. On the 19th April night, at 2 a.m., I received a call from the ward boy, making me rush to the ICU to find Ma's life signs slipping away!! The doctor on duty (Dr. Shonali) was trying her best and said to me: *"Dawa nahi dua ki zaroorat hai."* I stood silently, desperately looking at the monitor blip through the life support signs.

Even after two hours, her condition remained the same. That early morning Dr. Sanjeev Arora jumped into action. The entire day he stayed with Ma, ignoring the fact that it was a Sunday, his day off and sacrificing even his sister's engagement.

His priority lay in saving my mother's life, in the true sense of the word! Late afternoon, the vital stats came under control – it was a triumphant moment for all! Such was the dedication of oncology team!

With Baba, we had been witness to the utmost care Dr. Arun Verma took in the Radiation Department. Initially there was a confusion with the reports, whereby it was concluded that the cancer had spread to the nodes. The course of action was chalked out in a specific manner. But later, one of the radiologists countered the prognosis and Dr. Anand was called in for a review. After MRI and other tests, it turned out to be tuberculosis. The cancer was localised to the organ and had not spread. This was comforting and the actual treatment began. The whole course went quite smoothly and was hassle-free. Post-treatment results were extremely good and Baba is happy!

As kids, we cannot speak for Baba-Ma's emotions during the whole journey till remission, but we have seen the pain/ fear/ anticipation/ depression etched on their faces...never expressed vocally but endured silently!

It is one point in life when you feel the body weight in a literal sense. The bones and muscles no longer support you; the eyes fail, calling for cataract operation; the chemotherapy and radiation cause havoc to the digestive and excretory systems; you feel nauseous and dizzy all the time; the immune system is compromised as a result of which you are packed inside a sterile room, like new-born babies (*sans the joy*); you are dependent on maids/nurses/home-care folks, who are clocking 24/7; so called relatives and friends flood you with phone calls but prove of very little actual help; money flows down the drain, burning holes in your pocket; every time you go for a clinical test, your heart beat accelerates and you keep praying to God (*to give a good report*); any small parameter variance buzzes as an alarm (maybe false) – whether the cancer is back or not!

Is this really living? A million-dollar question indeed!

Not to mention the impact on the surrounding family members, who have to deal with daily nitty-gritties yet who continue to attend to the daily chores of family/school/office/household activities. But we believed that focus and determination proved to be the key. None of us could bring ourselves to accept the fact that *Death was knocking at the door*. We told ourselves that this was another medical issue which could be resolved by the best hands in Max Hospital team and network. We focused on the tiniest of the details and started taking baby steps towards recovery.

Nobody in the house ever discussed about

cancer in front of Baba-Ma; the discussions were regular ones... just like in any other normal household. We made them feel that 'it's okay, you will get through, don't worry'. We discussed movies and favourite TV serials; books, magazines and favourite authors; about our daily life stories at office, school, home. They played cards, celebrated birthdays and festivities with us, guided their grandchildren with maths and physics (they loved to solve challenging problems always); and when they felt better, they accompanied us to tours and travels to the mountains and green valleys.

Though at the back of the mind the *de- mentor* lurked, but we kept our windows (sic mind!) shut. Throughout the turbulent sail, our constant pole star was Dr. Meenu Walia and her oncology team. Every time we bugged her with our problems, she listened patiently and assured us with her innovative treatment plans and an ever-smiling face. Words have great power and her advice gave us immense strength to navigate through the dark alleys and finally pull out of it like a miracle! Her treatment procedure was excellent with minimal side effects and pain. She has been a brilliant researcher, an extremely considerate and kind doctor, always helping and her calm composure was a soothing balm to the ailing mind. Words fall short to describe her humane angle. She guided us through different steps in the cancer treatment and provided effective referral to other specialists at Max Hospital for all other ailments which proved quite helpful in managing holistic health (such as: cardio/ pulmonology/ urology/ radiation therapy/ neurology/ orthopaedics).

Today we are whole-heartedly indebted to Dr. Harit Chaturvedi too. He was our saviour and gladiator, who fought so well through the complex surgery. His expert hands eliminated all the marks and roots from within and Ma healed beautifully thereafter. A true cancer specialist in oncology surgery and best in Delhi/NCR! Timely referral by him to Dr. Meenu Walia for chemotherapy at the onset and subsequently when CA 125 dropped from 4795 (April 2014) to 15 (Sept. 2016). Dr. Meenu Walia referred the case back to Dr. Harit Chaturvedi for surgery and he executed it promptly, without any loss of time and in an excellent manner. Hats off to his team!

We remember staring at the nine jars (containing different body organs that had been removed) which were wheeled on a table from the OT, after six-and-a-half hours of surgery. The incision mark went all the way down, from the chest to the lower abdomen, like a post-mortem subject (*only in this case, she was our Ma and very much kicking*). A horrifying sight but much needed. Post care was tough but Ma did well and started shining like new within two-and-a-half months!

In a similar manner, Dr. Meenu Walia, timely referred Baba's case for radiation therapy, which helped to tackle the disease. We are sincerely grateful to Dr. Arun Verma for taking personal care during treatment period and at the OPD too.

We opted for home care services at Max and had a very good experience. They are professionals and took good care of the patient.

The last few years have been a game changer for me too – spending multiple years in the world of terminal disease wards where I discovered the meaning of LIFE in a very different way. It cannot be explained, but experienced only. So, no sermons here. We believe that there are only two days in the year that nothing can be done – one is called 'yesterday' and the other is called 'tomorrow', so today is the right day to love, believe, do and mostly LIVE. In everyone's life...before the best friends, spouse and everyone else in between, the first and arguably the most important relationship is the one with your parents. As kids, we are trying to keep that up!

Life has transitioned multifold before and after cancer...

Earlier, Baba remained busy with his engineering job and after retirement, he had taken up the role of HoD for the regional engineering college. Ma engaged herself with her mathematics teaching job and tutored many students after retirement. She also ran the huge household extremely efficiently.

Now, they spend 100 per cent of their time in each other's company, relishing each and every droplet of life, cherishing every sweet moment with unbound joy. They are celebrating their 50th golden anniversary together this year and we are all ecstatic with happiness and the flow of love that we experience each day in their company.

A few words from Baba and Ma: To overcome this disease, which is so expensive, we pray to God that even our deadliest enemies (even if they exist) should not suffer from cancer. You have faced many challenges in life and I have seen you fight and come out on top. This cancer is no different. You are fighters and I know you will come out on top as always.

To quote Robert Frost, 'Stopping by Woods on a Snowy Evening':

"The woods are lovely, dark and deep,
But I have promises to keep,
And miles to go before I sleep,
And miles to go before I sleep."

Ms. Saswati Sarkar
(Daughter)
Date: 2021

Warrior - 20

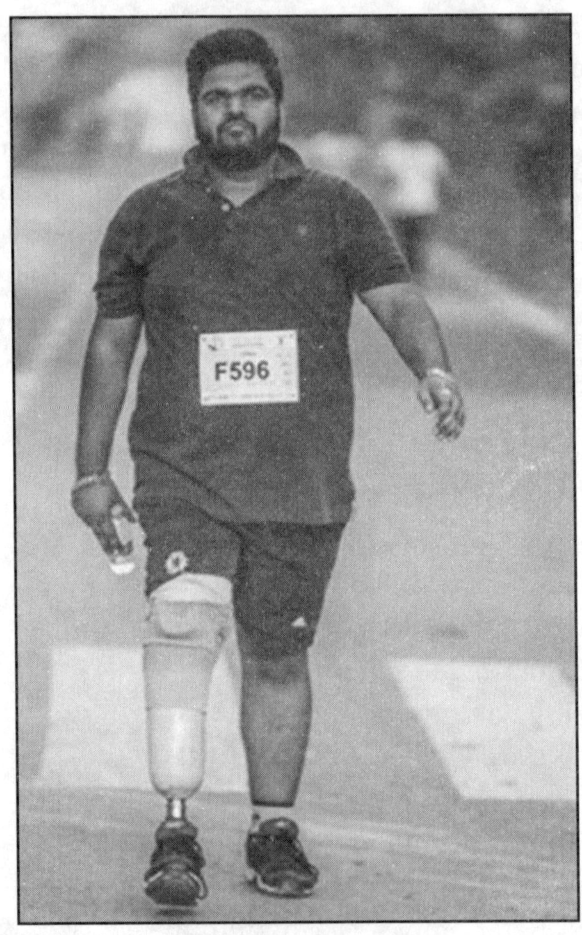

Hunny Kapoor
Diagnosed – 2015

मुझमें और किस्मत में हर बार बस यही जंग रही,
मैं उसके फैसलों से तंग वो मेरे हौंसलों से दंग रही!

A synovial sarcoma survivor and an amputee aged 26 years; I'm Hunny Kapoor, a motivational speaker, awardee, rider and a marathoner. What differentiates us among all is how we react to situations in life. I was leading a normal teenager's life, pursuing Maths (H) from Delhi University. Being an enthusiast, I used to give home tuitions, volunteered in NGOs, working part time in an MNC. I was trying to make my own space and luck in Delhi, Panipat being my hometown.

I lost equilibrium after four-and-a-half years of my journey in the capital and was diagnosed with sarcomatic cancer in right ankle, in March 2015. At the age of dating a girl, I was fixing appointments with doctors. My studies got affected and life turned upside down. Those were the most terrible moments of my life. In the beginning I wasn't able to accept the truth and hid it from my family for two days. I felt so burdened, unable to understand why it was happening with me and the troubling question, 'What's next?'

I can't remember how many times I tried to end my life. But my story in God's book wasn't finished yet. Anyhow, collecting my guts, I faced my parents about the situation. The tears in their eyes hit me hard but became my strength as I consoled myself maybe I can end everything with a full stop on my life but I've no right to put my parent's 22 years' investment on stake. Every single moment I tried to find a reason to blame this on. Couldn't find one!

Later on, doctors suggested that either I can save my life or my foot. I then made a tough choice. It took a week to convince my family to choose amputation as there was no better cure. Luckily, I got in touch with the Singapore Cancer Society and consulted them. I finally chose to fall in the category of 3 per cent of Indian population. I went under a series of surgeries. Everyone anticipated I would be completely bedridden and stuck to a wheelchair for life.

After my amputation, the scenario changed. My parents became more conscious of my activities. I lost all that I had gained but what I never lost was my confidence and will power. After all, a hero is not made of situations; he's the one who moulds them.

I practiced walking in prosthetics and maintained the pace of my life as far as possible. It's been four-and-a-half years since the amputation, I ride, commute on public transport, I swim and hit the gym daily. I'm pursuing graduation again, working in a private firm, interning as a campus ambassador, volunteering as a brand ambassador and as a business outreach with different organisations. I've been to open microphone and storytelling platforms, mental health seminars, workshops for specially-abled, been to events as a motivational speaker and I am a part of Human Library, Delhi as a 'human book'. I completed 20 marathons of 5 kms and 10th marathon of 10 Kms. Recently, my story was shared in the form of a motivational short film crossing 4.4 million views! https://www.youtube.com/watch?v=i5FOx1ub8c8. I was the core team member for Dance for Kindness, New Delhi, 2018 in November, covering 120 cities, 50 countries with over 20,000 participants. I was lucky enough to find a person who was aware of my story and the ups and downs – my partner. I've been awarded at different platforms and felicitated for the work I've done, breaking the stereotypes at being a role model.

So, cancer put a comma to my life but, not a full stop. It made me a fighter and I realised who Hunny Kapoor was. In the end, I am who I am because of my family and friends. Now that I am a survivor, I meet new people with the aim to create cancer awareness and make everyone realise that if I, despite all the odds, can do all this, then what's your excuse for not doing something....

Warrior - 21

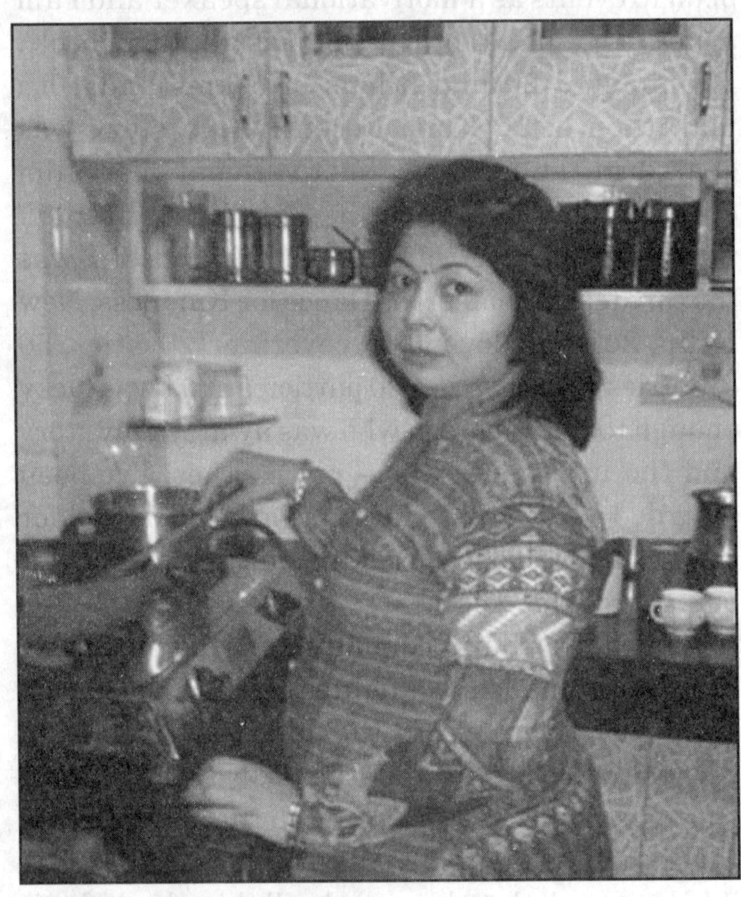

Tanisha Gaurav
Diagnosed – 2014

My name is Tanisha Gaurav and I am a patient of CML (chronic myelogenous leukaemia). In 2013, I was admitted to hospital for my second delivery. After four days, I developed a hard cough and the doctor advised a complete blood work. In my test results, TLC (total leukocyte count) was highly elevated and the doctor suspected blood cancer. I was in denial as to how a simple cold could be related to cancer. I repeated my tests in a different lab and the results came back the same. After the confirmation of my diagnosis of CML, I was totally emotionally drained. I was extremely worried about my new-born child, who was only nine-days old by then. He was so unfortunate not to have been nursed by me. I was crying the whole day as I felt I had lost life and had only a few days to live.

My treating doctor advised me to consult Dr. Meenu Walia. Right from the first consultation, she gave me a fresh lease of life through guidance and worthwhile counselling. She made me believe that CML was a curable cancer and there was nothing to worry about. She advised me routine medications and relevant investigations with proper follow-up.

For me she was like a second God and with full faith, I started treatment. She was there for my queries and my consolations. I was so lucky to have Dr. Walia in my cancer journey as she supported me on all aspects of my life. Even my family, especially my husband, helped me sail through this battle against blood cancer. Now I am on medications and regular follow-up and doing great with my children and my family.

Warrior - 22

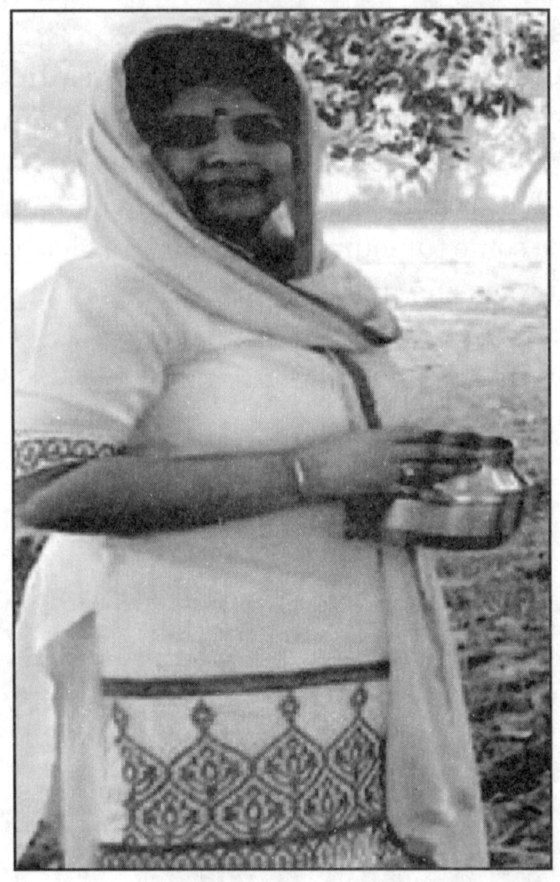

Jaya Chhonkar
Diagnosed – 2016

My journey with ovarian cancer started when I was suffering from stomach infection and bloating and this was in January 2016. I consulted my doctor, who advised me to undertake a routine ultrasound.

During the ultrasound, the radiologist discovered multiple cysts and fluid accumulation in my abdomen. Subsequently I was advised CT scan. The result of the CT scan was same and showed some tumours. On the basis of biopsy, I was diagnosed as having ovarian cancer, which was at Stage III. I was told that I had only ten months to survive. The feeling of imminent death was really painful.

I was admitted at Max Hospital under the supervision of Dr. Harit and Dr. Meenu Walia. I was totally disheartened and my perpetual thought was, 'Oh my God! Why have you chosen me to suffer?' As my mother had expired from the same disease and I had witnessed how much pain she had undergone, I was really worried about going through the same. But by God's grace, slowly and gradually, while visiting my doctors, I was able to regain my mental strength and confidence.

During the treatment, it was difficult to bear the pain after surgery and the endless nausea and vomiting after chemotherapy. My confidence was shattered, not only due to the pain which was unbearable, but also due to worry over the recurring expenses.

My family, my team of doctors and my friends stood by me in my darkest hours, trying to keep me motivated and encouraged. As I had been a social worker, the people I had helped earlier in their difficult times, told me that they prayed for my recovery and they also visited me, keeping me in good humour. It was a surprise package for me and I decided that it was all due to the good work I had done that life was repaying me in its own way.

I can't name a single person but it was the combined effort of many that saved my life. To be specific, I would like to thank my In-laws who took over the charge of running my home so that they could take proper care of my kids and husband. My husband, who always stood by me with a smile on his face, kept me happy. My social acquaintances prayed for me.

Last but not the least, I am grateful to my doctors, especially Dr Harit, who was available 24 hours for me; Dr Sanjeev, Dr Alok and Dr Geeta who persistently gave me the strength to recover; and Dr Meenu Walia, who helped me recover from pre- and post-chemotherapy. I am really thankful to all of them. I feel like I have been reborn again in my second life.

During this battle I learned that all you have to do is be mentally strong, keep yourself cool and positive and pray to the Almighty. I have also discovered that in my second life, I have become more humble and I am ready to do my social work with greater vigour and energy. After all, I owe my life to others now.

□

Conclusion

What have we seen; what have we learnt!!!

We realize the importance of being on land, after sailing a rough sea. When we have bargained for life, then we realize the beauty of each and every moment that passes by. Trust and love with the relatives and friends seem to have multiplied manifolds. Every greet and every bye seems special. Isn't this new life not worth enjoying?

You may have 101 grudges from your own life, but there will be 1000 others who might be dreaming to have the life you live.

A child on a farm sees an airplane and wishes to fly, whereas the pilot sees the farmhouse and dreams of returning home!

That's life... which comes with infinite perspectives and never ending possibilities! The only lesson that I have learnt about life is that... it goes on...

I will conclude with the following message for my readers:

"I Can...

...I will"

What mind doesnot know, eyes cannot see...

Knowledge Boosters for you!

A Cancer Battle Plan by Anne E. Frahm with David J. Frahm published by Jeremy P. Tarcher/Putnam, a member of Penguin Putnam Inc., New York, USA

Beating Cancer with Nutrition by Patrick Quillin with Noreen Quillin; published by Nutrition Times Pres Inc., Tulsa. Oklahoma, USA

Boundless Energy: The Complete Mind-Body Program Overcoming Fatigue by Deepak Chopra, published by RI:ER, an imprint of Ebury Press, Random House, London, UK

Buddha in Daily Life by Richard Causton., published by Rider, an imprint of Ebury Press, Random House, London, UK **Cancer Made Me** by Kasthuri Sreenivasans, published by Bharatiya Vidya Bhavan, Bombay, India

Cancer Talk by Selma R. Schimmel with Barry Fox., published by Broadway Books, a division of Random House, Inc. New York USA

Celebration of the Cells: Letters from a Cancer Survivor by R.M. Lala; published in Viking by Penguin Books India (P) Ltd., New Delhi, India

Chemotherapy and You: A Guide to Seit-he Treatment. Produced by National Cancer institute USA.

Courage and Contentment by Gurumayi Published by SYDA Foundation, New York, USA.

Creating Health by Deepak Chopra. Published by Thomsons, an imprint of Harper Collins Publishers, London UK.

Cultivating a Daily Meditation by Tenzin Gyatso. by the Library of Tibetan Works and Archives, Dharamsala India

Defeat the Dragon: Cure of Dreaded Diseases with Acupressure by Devendra Vora. Published by Navneet; Publications (India) Limited, Mumbai, India.

Eating Hints. Produced by National Cancer Institute Maryland, USA.

Foods that Heal: The Natural Way to Good Health by H.K. Bakhru. Published by Orient Paperbacks, a division of Vision Books Pvt. Ltd., Delhi, India.

Getting Well Again by O Carl Simonton, Stephanie Mathews-Simonton and James L. Creighton. Published by Bantam Books, a division of Bantam Doubleday, Dell Publishing Group Inc, New York, USA

Heal Your Body by Lousie L. Hay; published by Full Circle Publishing, New Delhi, India

Healing Emotions: Conversations with the Dalai Lama on Mindfulness, Emotions and Health. Edited by Damei Coleman; published by Shambhala Publications, Inc., Boston. USA

Health Through Balance: An Introduction to Tibetan Medicine by Dr. Yeshi Donden; edited and translated by Jeffery Hopkins published by Motilal Banarsidass Publishers Private Limited, Delhi.

Our Daily Bread by Dr. 'William Scott Literature for RBC Ministries, Chennai, India"

Principles of Ayurveda by Anne Green; Published by T. an imprint of Harper Collins Publishers, London UK

'Quantum Healing: Exploring the Frontiers of Mind/Body Medicine by Deepak Chopra; published by Bantam Books, New York, USA a division of Bantam Doubleday, Dell Publishing Group Inc. USA.

Six Months to Live: Learning from a Young Man With Cancer by Daniel Hallock; published by The plough Publishing House of The Bruderhof Foundation, Sussex, UK

Taking Time; prepared by the Office of Cancer Communications, National Cancer Institute, Maryland, USA

The Beginner's Guide to Zen Buddhism by Jean Smith, published by Bell Tower, a member of the Crown Publishing Group, Random House, Inc., New York, USA

The Healing Family: The Simonton Approach for Families Facing Illness by Stephanie Mathews-Sim on; published by Bantam Books, a division of Transworld Publishers Limited, London, UK

The Joy of Loving: A Guide to Daily Living with Mother Teresa. Compiled by Jaya Chaliha and Edward Le Joly., published in Viking by Penguin Books India (P) Ltd., New Delhi, India

The Joy of Reiki by Nalin Nirula and Renoo Nirula, published by Full Circle Publishing, New Delhi, India

The Path to Tranquility: Daily Meditations; edited by Renuka Singh. Published in Viking by Penguin Books India (P) Ltd., New Delhi, India

The Tibetan Book of Living and Dying by Sogyal Rinpoche published by Rider, an imprint of The Random House Group Limited, London, UK

Understanding Cancer of the Lung produced by the Queensland Cancer Fund, Australia

Understanding Emotions: produced by the National Cancer Institute, Maryland, USA

Understanding Nutrition; produced by the Queensland Cancer Fund, Australia

You Can Heal Your Life by Louise L Hay; published by full Circle Publishing, New Delhi, India

Important Websites

www.acor.org

www.cancer.org

www.cancercareinc.og

www.cancerguide.org

www.cancerhopenetwork.org

www.mskcc.org

www.nccn.org

www.ncinih.gov

www.oncolink.upenn.edu

www.breastcancer.about.com

www.nabco.org

www.ntlbcc.org

Brain Cancer

www.abta.org

Cervical Cancer

www.cervicalheathsorg

www.vulvarpainfoundaton.org

Leukemia

www.leukemia.org

Lung Cancer

www.alcase.org

www.lungusa.org

Prostate Cancer

www.afud.org

www.capcure.org

□

About the Author

Dr. (Prof.) Meenu Walia is a renowned medical oncologist practising in the National Capital Region of India. She has been dedicated to serving cancer patients for about three decades and continues to do so with full conviction. She started her journey as a Jr. Resident at Ram Manohar Lohia Hospital, New Delhi and currently spearheads the Department of Medical Oncology & Hematology at Max Super Speciality Hospital (Patparganj, Vaishali and Noida). She has the credit of being the first DNB medical oncologist of India.

On her professional front, Dr. Walia has a legacy par excellence. She believes in the principle of 'patient first' and has massively contributed towards uplifting patient care in her organisation. She is actively involved in clinical cancer research

About the Author

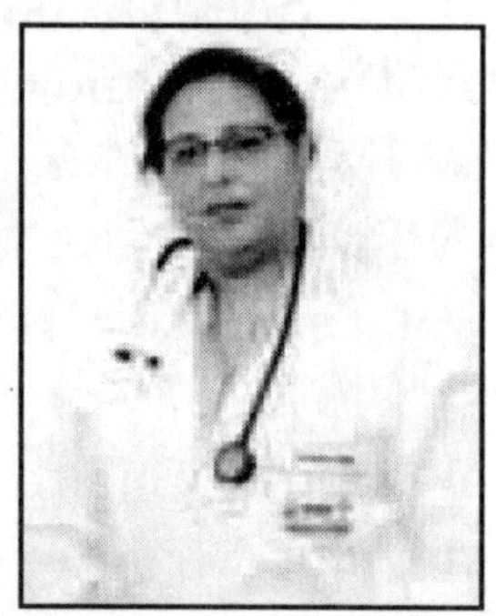

Dr. (Prof.) Meenu Walia is a renowned medical oncologist practicing in the National Capital Region of India. She has been dedicated to serving cancer patients for about three decades and continues to do so with full conviction. She started her journey as a Jr. Resident at Ram Manohar Lohia Hospital, New Delhi and currently spearheads the Department of Medical Oncology & Hematology at Max Super Speciality Hospital (Patparganj, Vaishali and Noida). She has the credit of being the first DNB medical oncologist of India.

On her professional front, Dr. Walia has a legacy par excellence. She believes in the principle of 'patient first' and has massively contributed towards uplifting patient care in her organisation. She is actively involved in clinical cancer research at global level and is the principal investigator in various global oncology research. She has been a part of more than 15 major global clinical trials. She is a teacher for the DNB medical oncology students. She is also a reviewer of medical journals, such as *Journal of Indian Academy of Clinical Medicine* and has authored chapters in several reputed books in her field of subject.

She has been decorated with the Bharat Jyoti Award and Certificate of Medical Excellence by IMA multiple times. She has been felicitated by President of India, Shri Ram Nath Kovind, as well as awarded the 'Inspiring Healthcare Leaders — Dronacharya Award', by the Hon'ble Minister of State for Health & Family Welfare, Government of India, Shri Ashwini Kumar Choubey. She has been conferred the 'Certificate of Excellence' in recognition of her exemplary work and dedication in the field of healthcare at the National Healthcare Conclave by (late) Shri Anant Kumar, Former Union Minister of Parliamentary Affairs.

She has been featured in '*Women of Wonder*' campaign by Radio Amity and Amity School of Communications. She has been felicitated with 'Most Influential Women of 2021' Award by Smt. Meenakshi Lekhi, Minister of State for External Affairs and national spokesperson of BJP. She has been conferred the 'Nari Astitva Award, 2021' and awarded the Lifetime Achievement Award by His

Excellency Moe Kyaw Aung, Ambassador of Myanmar to India at the Crown Global Awards, 2021. She has also been felicitated with the 6th International Healthcare Award.

Despite being a busy practitioner in her field, Dr. Walia is extremely active in working towards the welfare and supporting cancer patients, caregivers and NGOs in the field. She is a founder member and actively involved in development of support groups for cancer patients. Dr. Meenu Walia is also a TEDx speaker and her talk, 'How to Turnaround your Cancer Journey', has motivated several cancer patients.